Women's Mental Health

Editors

SUSAN G. KORNSTEIN
ANITA H. CLAYTON

MEDICAL CLINICS OF NORTH AMERICA

www.medical.theclinics.com

Consulting Editor
BIMAL H. ASHAR

July 2019 • Volume 103 • Number 4

ELSEVIER

1600 John F. Kennedy Boulevard • Suite 1800 • Philadelphia, Pennsylvania, 19103-2899

http://www.theclinics.com

MEDICAL CLINICS OF NORTH AMERICA Volume 103, Number 4
July 2019 ISSN 0025-7125, ISBN-13: 978-0-323-71345-0

Editor: Jessica McCool
Developmental Editor: Kristen Helm

Medical Clinics of North America (ISSN 0025-7125) is published bimonthly by Elsevier Inc., 360 Park Avenue South, New York, NY 10010-1710. Months of publication are January, March, May, July, September, and November. Business and editorial offices: 1600 John F. Kennedy Boulevard, Suite 1800, Philadelphia, PA 19103-2899. Periodicals postage paid at New York, NY, and additional mailing offices. Subscription prices are USD $284.00 per year (US individuals), $611.00 per year (US institutions), $100.00 per year (US Students), $353.00 per year (Canadian individuals), $794.00 per year (Canadian institutions), $200.00 per year (Canadian and foreign students), $406.00 per year (foreign individuals), and $794.00 per year (foreign institutions). To receive student/resident rate, orders must be accompanied by name of affiliated institution, date of term, and the signature of program/residency coordinator on institution letterhead. Orders will be billed at individual rate until proof of status is received. Foreign air speed delivery is included in all Clinics' subscription prices. All prices are subject to change without notice. **POSTMASTER:** Send address changes to *Medical Clinics of North America*, Elsevier Health Sciences Division, Subscription Customer Service, 3251 Riverport Lane, Maryland Heights, MO 63043. **Customer Service: Telephone: 1-800-654-2452** (U.S. and Canada); **1-314-447-8871** (outside U.S. and Canada). **Fax: 314-447-8029. E-mail: journalscustomerserviceusa@elsevier.com** (for print support); **journalsonlinesupport-usa@elsevier.com** (for online support).

Reprints. For copies of 100 or more of articles in this publication, please contact the Commercial Reprints Department, Elsevier Inc., 360 Park Avenue South, New York, NY 10010-1710. Tel.: 212-633-3874; Fax: 212-633-3820; E-mail: reprints@elsevier.com.

Medical Clinics of North America is also published in Spanish by McGraw-Hill Interamericana Editores S. A., P.O. Box 5-237, 06500 Mexico, D.F., Mexico.

Medical Clinics of North America is covered in *MEDLINE/PubMed (Index Medicus), Current Contents, ASCA, Excerpta Medica, Science Citation Index, and ISI/BIOMED.*

Printed in the United States of America.

PROGRAM OBJECTIVE

The goal of the *Medical Clinics of North America* is to keep practicing physicians up to date with current clinical practice by providing timely articles reviewing the state of the art in patient care.

TARGET AUDIENCE

All practicing physicians and other healthcare professionals.

LEARNING OBJECTIVES

Upon completion of this activity, participants will be able to:

1. Review premenstrual dysphoric disorder
2. Discuss updates on reproductive rights and women's mental health
3. Recognize updates on mental health aspects of intimate partner violence and in sexual minority and transgender women

ACCREDITATION

The Elsevier Office of Continuing Medical Education (EOCME) is accredited by the Accreditation Council for Continuing Medical Education (ACCME) to provide continuing medical education for physicians.

The EOCME designates this enduring material for a maximum of 15 *AMA PRA Category 1 Credit*(s)™. Physicians should claim only the credit commensurate with the extent of their participation in the activity.

All other healthcare professionals requesting continuing education credit for this enduring material will be issued a certificate of participation.

DISCLOSURE OF CONFLICTS OF INTEREST

The EOCME assesses conflict of interest with its instructors, faculty, planners, and other individuals who are in a position to control the content of CME activities. All relevant conflicts of interest that are identified are thoroughly vetted by EOCME for fair balance, scientific objectivity, and patient care recommendations. EOCME is committed to providing its learners with CME activities that promote improvements or quality in healthcare and not a specific proprietary business or a commercial interest.

The planning committee, staff, authors and editors listed below have identified no financial relationships or relationships to products or devices they or their spouse/life partner have with commercial interest related to the content of this CME activity:
Bimal H. Ashar, MD, MBA, FACP; Nassima Ait-Daoud, MD; Margaret Altemus, MD; Pooja Amin, BS, MD; Leah S. Casuto, MD; Todd M. Derreberry, MD; Laura Erickson-Schroth, MD, MA; Kristen Helm; Suzanne Holroyd, MD; Christopher P. Holstege, MD; Surbhi Khanna, MD; Alison Kemp; Teresa Lanza di Scalea, MD, PhD; Jessica McCool; Nicole Mori, RN, BSN, APRN-BC; Teri Pearlstein, MD; Julie K. Schulman, MD; Sana Sharma, MD; Nada Logan Stotland, MD, MPH; Jeyanthi Surendrakumar; Elia Margarita Valladares Juarez, MD.

The planning committee, staff, authors and editors listed below have identified financial relationships or relationships to products or devices they or their spouse/life partner have with commercial interest related to the content of this CME activity:
Anita H. Clayton, MD: receives research support from Endoceutics, Inc. and Janssen Pharmaceuticals, Inc.; is a consultant/advisor for ACADIA Pharmaceuticals Inc., Alkermes, Allergan, AMAG Pharmaceuticals, Fabre-Kramer Pharmaceuticals, Inc., Lundbeck, Otsuka America Pharmaceutical, Inc., Palatin Technologies, Inc., Sprout Pharmaceuticals, Inc.; is a consultant/advisor for and receives research support from Sage Therapeutics, Inc. and Takeda Pharmaceutical Company Limited; receives royalties from Penguin Random House LLC and Guilford Press; is a consultant/advisor and owns stock in S1 Biopharma, Inc.; owns stock in Euthymics Bioscience, Inc.
Anna I. Guerdjikova, PhD, LISW: is a consultant/advisor for Avanir Pharmaceuticals, Inc and Bracket
Susan G. Korstein, MD: is a consultant/advisor Eli Lilly and Company, Sunovion Pharmaceuticals Inc., Allergan, and ACADIA Pharmaceuticals Inc.; receives research support from Pfizer Inc., Marinus Pharmaceuticals, Inc., Takeda Pharmaceutical Company Limited, and Palatin Technologies, Inc.
Susan L. McElroy, MD: is a consultant/advisor for Bracket, F. Hoffmann-La Roche Ltd., Mitsubishi Tanabe Pharma America, and Opiant Pharmaceuticals; is a consultant/advisor for and receives research support from Avanir Pharmaceuticals, Inc., Allergan, Myriad Genetics, Inc., Shire, and Sunovion Pharmaceuticals Inc.; receives research support from Azevan Pharmaceuticals, Inc., Brainsway, Medibio Limited, Neurocrine Biosciences, Inc., and Novo Nordisk; holds a patent with Johnson & Johnson Services, Inc.
Jennifer L. Payne, MD: is a consultant/advisor for AstraZeneca, Johnson & Johnson Services, Inc, Eli Lilly and Company, and Pfizer Inc. Dr. Payne also receives research support from Sage Therapeutics, Inc.

Claudio N. Soares, MD, PhD, FRCPC, MBA: is a consultant for Pfizer Inc., Sunovion Pharmaceuticals Inc, Merck Sharp & Dohme Corp, Otsuka Pharmaceutical Co., Ltd., Servier Pharmaceuticals LLC., and Lundbeck.

Donna Eileen Stewart, CM, MD, FRCPC: receives royalties from UpToDate, Inc. and is a consultant/advisor for Eli Lilly and Company

Simone Natalie Vigod, MD, MSc, FRCPC: receives royalties from UpToDate, Inc.

UNAPPROVED/OFF-LABEL USE DISCLOSURE

The EOCME requires CME faculty to disclose to the participants;

1. When products or procedures being discussed are off-label, unlabelled, experimental, and/or investigational (not US Food and Drug Administration [FDA] approved); and
2. Any limitations on the information presented, such as data that are preliminary or that represent ongoing research, interim analyses, and/or unsupported opinions. Faculty may discuss information about pharmaceutical agents that is outside of FDA-approved labelling. This information is intended solely for CME and is not intended to promote off-label use of these medications. If you have any questions, contact the medical affairs department of the manufacturer for the most recent prescribing information.

TO ENROLL

To enroll in the *Medical Clinics of North America* Continuing Medical Education program, call customer service at 1-800-654-2452 or sign up online at http://www.theclinics.com/home/cme. The CME program is available to subscribers for an additional annual fee of USD $300.90.

METHOD OF PARTICIPATION

In order to claim credit, participants must complete the following;

1. Complete enrolment as indicated above.
2. Read the activity.
3. Complete the CME Test and Evaluation. Participants must achieve a score of 70% on the test. All CME Tests and Evaluations must be completed online.

CME INQUIRIES/SPECIAL NEEDS

For all CME inquiries or special needs, please contact elsevierCME@elsevier.com.

MEDICAL CLINICS OF NORTH AMERICA

FORTHCOMING ISSUES

September 2019
Cardiac Arrhythmias: A Compendium
Otto Costantini, *Editor*

November 2019
Genetics and Precision Medicine
Howard P. Levy, *Editor*

January 2020
Allergy and Immunology for the Internist
Anne M. Ditto, *Editor*

RECENT ISSUES

May 2019
Pulmonary Disease
Ali I. Musani, *Editor*

March 2019
Neurology for the Non-Neurologist
Tracey A. Milligan, *Editor*

January 2019
Gastroenterology for the Internist
Kerry B. Dunbar, *Editor*

SERIES OF RELATED INTEREST

Primary Care: Clinics in Office Practice
Physician Assistant Clinics
Psychiatric Clinics of North America

Contributors

CONSULTING EDITOR

BIMAL H. ASHAR, MD, MBA, FACP
Associate Professor of Medicine, Division of General Internal Medicine, Johns Hopkins School of Medicine, Baltimore, Maryland, USA

EDITORS

SUSAN G. KORNSTEIN, MD
Professor, Department of Psychiatry and Institute for Women's Health, Virginia Commonwealth University, Virginia Commonwealth University, Richmond, Virginia, USA

ANITA H. CLAYTON, MD
David C. Wilson Professor and Chair, Department of Psychiatry and Neurobehavioral Sciences, Professor of Clinical Obstetrics & Gynecology, University of Virginia, Charlottesville, Virginia, USA

AUTHORS

NASSIMA AIT-DAOUD, MD
Associate Professor, Department of Psychiatry and Neurobehavioral Sciences, University of Virginia, Charlottesville, Virginia, USA

MARGARET ALTEMUS, MD
Associate Professor of Psychiatry, Yale School of Medicine, VA Connecticut Healthcare System, West Haven, Connecticut, USA

POOJA AMIN, BS, MD
Research Associate, Department of Psychiatry and Neurobehavioral Sciences, University of Virginia, Charlottesville, Virginia, USA

DEREK BLEVINS, MD
Department of Psychiatry and Neurobehavioral Sciences, University of Virginia, Charlottesville, Virginia, USA

LEAH S. CASUTO, MD
Lindner Center of HOPE, Mason, Ohio; Department of Psychiatry and Behavioral Neuroscience, University of Cincinnati College of Medicine, Cincinnati, Ohio, USA

ANITA H. CLAYTON, MD
David C. Wilson Professor and Chair, Department of Psychiatry and Neurobehavioral Sciences, Professor of Clinical Obstetrics & Gynecology, University of Virginia, Charlottesville, Virginia, USA

TODD M. DERREBERRY, MD
Assistant Professor of Psychiatry, Department of Psychiatry and Behavioral Medicine, Joan C. Edwards School of Medicine, Marshall University, Huntington, West Virginia, USA

TERESA LANZA DI SCALEA, MD, PhD
Attending Psychiatrist, Department of Psychiatry, Rhode Island Hospital and Miriam Hospital, Providence, Rhode Island, USA

LAURA ERICKSON-SCHROTH, MD, MA
Assistant Professor, Department of Psychiatry, Mount Sinai Beth Israel, New York, New York, USA

ANNA I. GUERDJIKOVA, PhD, LISW
Lindner Center of HOPE, Mason, Ohio; Department of Psychiatry and Behavioral Neuroscience, University of Cincinnati College of Medicine, Cincinnati, Ohio, USA

SUZANNE HOLROYD, MD
Professor and Chair of Psychiatry, Department of Psychiatry and Behavioral Medicine, Joan C. Edwards School of Medicine, Marshall University, Huntington, West Virginia, USA

CHRISTOPHER P. HOLSTEGE, MD
Professor, Division of Medical Toxicology, Department of Emergency Medicine, University of Virginia, Charlottesville, Virginia, USA

SURBHI KHANNA, MD
Department of Psychiatry and Neurobehavioral Sciences, University of Virginia, Charlottesville, Virginia, USA

SUSAN L. McELROY, MD
Lindner Center of HOPE, Mason, Ohio; Department of Psychiatry and Behavioral Neuroscience, University of Cincinnati College of Medicine, Cincinnati, Ohio, USA

NICOLE MORI, RN, MSN, APRN-BC
Lindner Center of HOPE, Mason, Ohio; Department of Psychiatry and Behavioral Neuroscience, University of Cincinnati College of Medicine, Cincinnati, Ohio, USA

JENNIFER L. PAYNE, MD
Associate Professor of Psychiatry, Johns Hopkins School of Medicine, Baltimore, Maryland, USA

TERI PEARLSTEIN, MD
Professor, Departments of Psychiatry and Human Behavior and Medicine, Alpert Medical School of Brown University, Director, Women's Behavioral Medicine, Women's Medicine Collaborative, Miriam Hospital, Providence, Rhode Island, USA

JULIE K. SCHULMAN, MD
Assistant Professor of Psychiatry, Department of Consultation-Liaison Psychiatry, Allen Hospital, New York, New York, USA

SANA SHARMA, MD
Department of Psychiatry and Neurobehavioral Sciences, University of Virginia, Charlottesville, Virginia, USA

CLAUDIO N. SOARES, MD, PhD, FRCPC, MBA
Professor, Department of Psychiatry, Queen's University School of Medicine, Executive Lead, Research and Innovation, Providence Care Hospital, Kingston, Ontario, Canada

DONNA EILEEN STEWART, CM, MD, FRCPC
University Professor, University of Toronto, Senior Scientist, Toronto General Hospital Research Institute, Research Head, Centre for Mental Health, University Health Network, Toronto, Ontario, Canada

NADA LOGAN STOTLAND, MD, MPH
Professor of Psychiatry, Rush University, Chicago, Illinois, USA

ELIA MARGARITA VALLADARES JUAREZ, MD
Assistant Professor, Department of Psychiatry and Neurobehavioral Sciences, University of Virginia Health System, Charlottesville, Virginia, USA

SIMONE NATALIE VIGOD, MD, MSc, FRCPC
Scientist, Women's College Hospital and Research Institute, Assistant Professor, University of Toronto, Toronto, Ontario, Canada

Contents

origins of these barriers, their nature, and their impact on mental health. The most controversial relationship is between induced abortion and mental health. Barriers, misinformation, and coercion affecting contraceptive, abortion, and pregnancy care are an ongoing danger to women's mental health and the well-being of their families. Mental health professionals are best qualified, and have an obligation, to know the facts, apply them, and provide accurate information to protect women's health.

Preface

Women's Mental Health: Progress and Realities

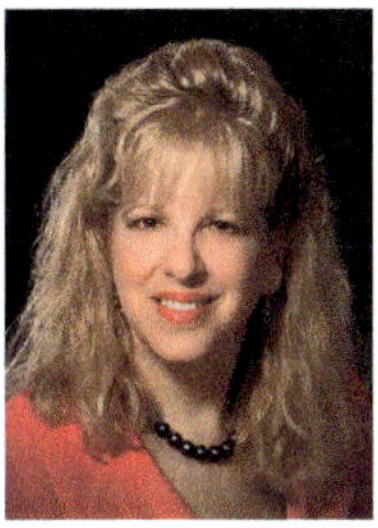 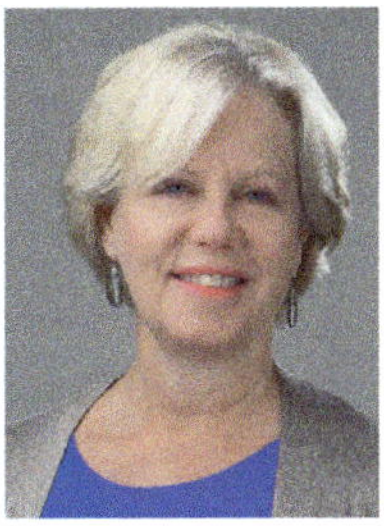

Susan G. Kornstein, MD Anita H. Clayton, MD
Editors

The field of women's mental health has grown tremendously over the past several decades. Some of the growth in this area has been related to a national focus on health care, with particular attention to conditions specific to women, sex and gender differences, and reproductive rights. Federal agencies have put policies in place about research requiring consideration of sex in study design, recruitment, and analysis, and clinicians have begun to implement aspects of personalized medicine, which may change for women across the life cycle. The knowledge base has grown considerably and has expanded into new areas, such as female sexual dysfunction, with the first medical treatment approved by the Food and Drug Administration (FDA) in 2015. Progress in the diagnostic classification of disorders in women is evident in the *Diagnostic and Statistical Manual of Mental Disorders* (Fifth Edition) (*DSM-5*), which for the first time includes premenstrual dysphoric disorder in the main text as well as the mood disorder specifier "with perinatal onset." New data regarding sex and gender differences in prevalence, cause, presentation, interventions, and response to treatment are impacting care of women and stimulating new research. A medication with a new mechanism of action (positive allosteric neuromodulator) and a unique treatment paradigm (brief intravenous infusion) with a specific indication for postpartum depression has just been approved. Organizations and conferences on women's mental health are increasing in number and providing more opportunities for clinicians and researchers to share their knowledge, such as the 8th World Congress on Women's Mental Health this year in Paris.

This issue begins with a summary by Margaret Altemus of the latest science concerning neuroendocrine networks and functionality. She discusses the developmental

Med Clin N Am 103 (2019) xv–xvii
https://doi.org/10.1016/j.mcna.2019.03.004
0025-7125/19/© 2019 Published by Elsevier Inc.

and cyclic changes in hormonal exposures in women that can impact brain function and mental health. This sets the stage for several articles related to reproductive mood disorders. Teresa Lanza di Scalea and Teri Pearlstein provide an overview of premenstrual dysphoric disorder; Jennifer Payne presents the newest guidelines for psychotropic use during pregnancy and breastfeeding, and Claudio Soares discusses the evaluation and treatment of depression related to the menopause transition.

A brand new diagnosis in the *DSM-5* is binge-eating disorder (BED), which is presented by Anna Guerdjikova, Nicole Mori, Leah Casuto, and Susan McElroy. BED is now recognized as the most common eating disorder, and the FDA recently approved the first medication for its treatment. Another area with exciting developments in the past several years is female sexual dysfunction, which is addressed by Anita Clayton and Elia Margarita Valladares Juarez.

The number of women becoming addicted to alcohol or drugs of abuse has significantly increased, and women have been disproportionately affected by the opioid epidemic. Nassima Ait-Daoud, Derek Blevins, Surbhi Khanna, Sana Sharma, Christopher Holstege, and Pooja Amin provide a comprehensive overview of gender considerations in the assessment and treatment of addiction.

Dementia is an increasing problem in women worldwide due to the higher prevalence in women than in men, the aging population, and the longer lifespan of women compared with men. Todd Derreberry and Suzanne Holroyd review the latest knowledge on sex and gender differences in Alzheimer disease and other dementias as well as the caregiving burden that affects many women.

Despite progress in achieving civil rights, sexual minority and transgender women face significant discrimination (eg, attempts to exclude transgender individuals from serving in the US military), harassment and violence (eg, mass shooting in the LGBTQ [lesbian, gay, bisexual, transgender, questioning, or queer] nightclub *Pulse* in Orlando, Florida in 2016), as well as increased rates of mental illness and substance use disorders. Julie Schulman and Laura Erickson-Schroth provide an introduction and recommendations for working with sexual minority and transgender women. Intimate partner violence (IPV) occurs in over one-third of American women. Donna Stewart and Simone Vigod discuss mental health aspects of IPV, including risk factors, sequelae, and management. The article by Nada Stotland discusses reproductive rights as essential to women's mental health. Although the World Health Organization proclaims access to reproductive health care as a basic human right, ongoing barriers, misinformation, and coercion affecting contraceptive, abortion, and pregnancy care pose a danger to the mental health and well-being of women and their families.

We are grateful to the authors for their outstanding contributions and to the publisher for allowing us this opportunity. We are confident that readers will find that the contents of this issue will greatly enhance their care of women patients.

Susan G. Kornstein, MD
Department of Psychiatry and
Institute for Women's Health
Virginia Commonwealth University
P.O. Box 980319
Virginia Commonwealth University
Richmond, VA 23298, USA

Anita H. Clayton, MD
Department of Psychiatry and
Neurobehavioral Sciences
University of Virginia
2955 Ivy Road
Northridge Suite 210
Charlottesville, VA 22093, USA

E-mail addresses:
susan.kornstein@vcuhealth.org (S.G. Kornstein)
AHC8V@hscmail.mcc.virginia.edu (A.H. Clayton)

Neuroendocrine Networks and Functionality

Margaret Altemus, MD

KEYWORDS

• Estrogen • Progesterone • Puberty • Lactation • Menopause • Menstrual cycle • Pregnancy

KEY POINTS

- Premenstrual symptoms most commonly include irritability, tension, mood lability, sleep changes, fatigue, increased appetite, and fluid retention, and are stimulated by luteal secretion of progesterone.
- During pregnancy, physiologic responses to stress are relatively suppressed but there is no reduction in rates of depression or other psychiatric disorders during pregnancy.
- After delivery, women are at increased risk for relapse or first episode of bipolar disorder. Women with antithyroid antibodies are at high risk for developing hyperthyroidism or hypothyroidism postpartum.
- The risk of major depression in increased in women compared with men from the onset of ovarian cycling at puberty until menopause, with the highest relative risk occurring in the years preceding menopause.

Women undergo developmental and cyclic changes in hormonal exposures that affect brain function and some aspects of mental health. The fluctuations in gonadal steroids and hypothalamic-pituitary-adrenal (HPA) axis regulation across the menstrual cycle and pregnancy are necessary for conception and gestation but also expose women to repeated and large perturbations of gonadal steroid and glucocorticoid responsive brain systems. In addition, the thyroid axis is at increased risk of dysregulation during and after pregnancy, which in turn increases risk for affective illness.

It is important to note that there are large individual differences in the activational effects of reproductive hormones on behavior. Although almost all women undergo the hormonal fluctuations related to menstruation, pregnancy, and menopause, few women (3%–5%) experience the intense perimenstrual negative affect that occurs in women with premenstrual dysphoric disorder (PMDD)[1] and, similarly, small subgroups of women experience postpartum or perimenopausal depression.[2,3] The

This article originally appeared in the *Psychiatric Clinics of North America*, Volume 40, Issue 2, June 2017.
The author has nothing to disclose.
VA Connecticut Health Care System, Women's Clinic, Building 2, Room 7-165, 950 Campbell Avenue, New Haven, CT 06516, USA
E-mail address: margaret.altemus@yale.edu

Med Clin N Am 103 (2019) 601–612
http://dx.doi.org/10.1016/j.mcna.2019.03.003
0025-7125/19/Published by Elsevier Inc.

bulk of research indicates that these subgroups of women experience the typical changes in levels of estrogen, progesterone, and other reproductive hormones but a suboptimal central nervous system response that leads to negative affect and maladaptive behaviors.[4,5] Both inherited genotype and developmental experiences likely contribute to these individual differences among women. Life experiences and cultural expectations clearly shape subjective experience, resiliency, and behavior. In addition, there is evidence that experience alters gene expression and contributes to biological changes in brain and physiology throughout the lifespan.[6] Finally, it can be difficult to tease apart the effect of hormonal changes associated with puberty, pregnancy, and menopause from the profound psychosocial changes that can accompany these life stages.

The onset of anxiety and affective disorders peaks during adolescence and early adulthood, with female patients being at significantly greater risk than male patients. Women have twice the lifetime rates of depression and most anxiety disorders.[7–10] The exceptions in term of sex ratio are obsessive compulsive disorder (OCD) and bipolar disorder, which have similar prevalence in men and women. However, even for these disorders, men and women have differences in disease presentation and course.[11–13] In addition to higher rates of affective disorders that meet full diagnostic criteria, subclinical anxiety and depression symptoms are also more common in women.[14,15] Sex differences in prevalence rates and symptom course of other psychiatric disorders are less clearly linked to adult hormonal fluctuations, with the exception of schizophrenia.

This article summarizes hormonal fluctuations in women across development and the associated impact on mental health.

PRENATAL

There are multiple organizational effects of gonadal steroid exposure during development.[16,17] In humans, exposure to fetal sex hormones starts at gestational week 7, at which point the male fetus begins to produce testosterone, resulting in differentiation of the male genitalia and sex differences in the brain and other tissues. Testosterone levels peak in the fetal serum in males between weeks 12 and 18 of pregnancy.[18] Immediately after birth, there is a second peak in testosterone in boys and a peak in estrogens in girls.[19] The testosterone levels of the male newborn are ten times higher than those of the female and this surge persists for 3 months after birth.[20] Lower amniotic fluid testosterone levels at midgestation (weeks 13–20) were associated with a negative response bias and less response to rewarding stimuli during a functional MRI task among boys studied between 8 to 11 years of age,[21] suggesting that the relatively greater levels of androgen exposure in utero may contribute to relative protection against depression later in life. Biologically determined sex differences can arise from effects of sex chromosome genes, independent of reproductive hormone exposure.[22–25] In addition, recent animal studies suggest that maternal and paternal stress that occurs even before conception can have differential effects in male and female offspring on depression and anxiety-related behaviors and stress-response regulation.[26,27] In humans, elevated levels of maternal depression and cortisol during pregnancy,[28,29] and elevated milk cortisol levels during lactation,[30] have been associated with more fearful and reactive behavior in female infants and children compared with male offspring.

CHILDHOOD

In contrast to major depression, which has an increased prevalence in girls beginning in midpuberty, the increased risk of anxiety and some anxiety disorders in girls begins in middle childhood.[31] Prepubertal girls have 2-fold higher rates of rates of separation anxiety, specific phobias, and social phobia than boys, pointing out mechanisms other than ovarian cycling contribute to increased rates of these anxiety disorders in women. In addition, the increased tendency to ruminate, a risk factor for major depression, emerges in girls by age 9, also before puberty.[32]

PUBERTY

Longitudinal studies have identified Tanner stage III, the start of ovarian cycling, when estrogen levels rise significantly, as the onset of increased rates of major depression in girls.[33] Longitudinal cohort studies suggest that low birth weight and being small for gestational age, evidence of a suboptimal in utero milieu and fetal stress, lead to relatively greater risk of depression in adolescent[34–36] and adult women[37] but not preadolescent girls.[35,36] Higher rates of interpersonal stress have been shown to partially mediate the increased prevalence of depression in girls after puberty.[38,39] After puberty, women experience major depression at roughly twice the rate of male patients until late middle age when women transition to menopause. The higher rates of generalized anxiety disorder and panic disorder in women also are not evident until adolescence.[40]

MENSTRUAL CYCLE

Although women with depression and anxiety disorders often report a worsening of chronic symptoms premenstrually,[41] another distinctive set of mood and physical symptoms can be associated with only the luteal phase of the menstrual cycle, including prominent emotional symptoms of irritability, tension, and mood lability, as well as physical symptoms of fluid retention, increased appetite, and fatigue. The distinct hormonal change in the luteal phase is secretion of progesterone by the corpus luteum, which begins at ovulation and falls to baseline during the last few days of the luteal phase, triggering the onset of menses (**Fig. 1**). Although mild symptoms are very common in the final days of the luteal phase, women with more severe symptoms that impair functioning and meet criteria for PMDD, often have symptoms lasting 5 to 7 days and as long as 14 days of the luteal phase. Women with PMDD do not seem to have abnormal levels of estrogen, progesterone, or other gonadal steroids across the cycle[42] but, instead, seem to be more reactive to luteal phase progesterone in terms of both mood and physical symptoms.[4] Experimental and treatment studies have shown that PMDD symptoms are relieved by elimination of ovulation and reproduced by exogenous progesterone administration.[4] However, progesterone receptor

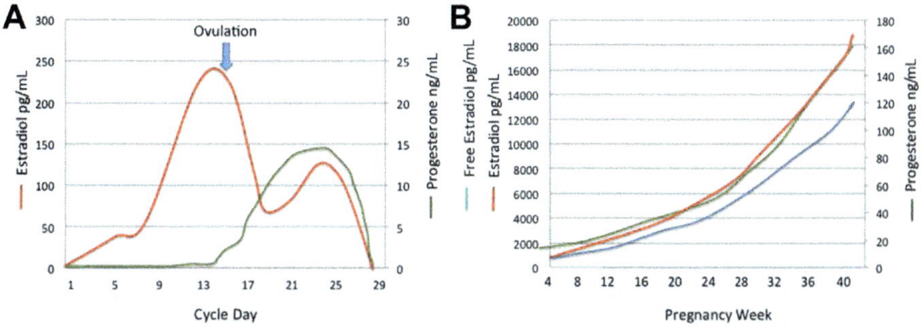

Fig. 1. Magnitude of estradiol and progesterone changes during (*A*) the menstrual cycle and (*B*) pregnancy.

blockade does not relieve symptoms,[43] indicating that symptoms are generated by a metabolite of progesterone, or progesterone acting through membrane effects or other nonclassic receptor mechanisms.

One distinctive feature of PMDD is the selective response to selective serotonin reuptake inhibitor (SSRI) and serotonin and norepinephrine reuptake inhibitor (SNRI) antidepressant agents, suggesting that this PMDD involves a vulnerability to dysregulation of serotonergic systems. Alternatively, the greater efficacy of SSRIs in PMDD may be due to SSRI induction of 3-alpha reductase,[44,45] the enzyme producing the anxiolytic metabolite allopregnanolone (3-alpha,5-alpha progesterone).[46] Women using cyclic hormonal contraceptives, who are unlikely to be ovulating, can report premenstrual syndrome with a similar pattern, intensity, and duration of symptoms that responds to SSRI treatment.[47]

Retrospective reports of women who meet full diagnostic criteria for PMDD indicate high comorbidity with major depression, bipolar disorder, seasonal affective disorder, and panic disorder.[48] However, this indication of shared vulnerability for PMDD and other affective disorders needs to be confirmed by controlled, prospective studies. It also remains to be determined whether PMDD is associated with an increased risk of depression during pregnancy or postpartum, when hormonal changes are much larger, more numerous, and more sustained (see **Fig. 1**).

There has been relatively little study of the effect of the menstrual cycle on bipolar symptoms but preliminary evidence suggests that women with bipolar disorder have increased rates of PMDD and approximately 50% of women with bipolar disorder report mood changes tied to their menstrual cycle, including, in some cases, manic symptoms at ovulation and premenstrually.[49] Women with social anxiety and OCD also often experience symptom exacerbation premenstrually.[50] However, rates of comorbid PMDD have not been carefully studied. The frequency of binge eating is also increased premenstrually.[51] Finally, a few experimental studies have demonstrated increased vulnerability to intrusive negative memories, when traumatic material is presented in the early luteal phase of the menstrual cycle compared with the follicular or late luteal phase.[52] In contrast, hospital admission for schizophrenia and schizophrenia symptom severity is highest in the perimenstrual and early follicular phase, when estrogen and progesterone levels are lowest.[53–55]

Because there are such clear sex differences in HPA axis regulation in rodents, and HPA axis regulation is often disturbed during depressive episodes, much attention has been focused on a causal role for sex differences in the HPA axis in generating sex differences in vulnerability to depression. However, sex differences in HPA axis regulation are much smaller and less consistent in humans than rodents.[56,57] Increased reactivity of the HPA axis and reduced sensitivity to glucocorticoid feedback can be demonstrated in the luteal phase of the menstrual cycle in humans following pharmacologic and stress challenges[58–60] but baseline levels of cortisol secretion are stable across the cycle. Of note, women with PMDD do not show this typical change in HPA axis regulation in the luteal phase, indicating that they have a different reaction to the luteal surge in progesterone.[59]

PREGNANCY

During pregnancy, women are exposed to very high circulating levels of multiple hormones produced by the placenta, including but not limited to estrogens, androgens, progesterone, allopregnanolone, prolactin, corticotropin-releasing hormone (CRH), and oxytocin. Cortisol levels are also very high, stimulated by placental CRH. Despite a rise in sex hormone–binding globulin and cortisol-binding globulin during pregnancy, the free fractions of these steroid hormones are elevated and cross the blood brain barrier. Less is known about central activity of reproductive peptide hormones during pregnancy but elevations in cerebrospinal fluid CRH and prolactin, and normal levels of cerebrospinal fluid oxytocin, have been documented during late pregnancy in humans.[61,62] After delivery, there is an abrupt drop in all of the hormones and peptides produced by the placenta.

It is arguable whether there is an increased risk of major depression in relation to pregnancy and childbirth, although the *Diagnostic and Statistical Manual for Mental Disorders*, 5th edition,[63] allows for the continued use of the peripartum onset specifier for occurrence of major depression in the third trimester and up to 4 weeks after childbirth. The heterogeneity of depression and of groups studied may obscure the true relationship between major depression and perinatal hormonal fluctuations. Of women who have major depression postpartum, approximately one-quarter have chronic depression, one-third have depression with onset during pregnancy, and only a little more than one-third have actual postpartum onset of depression.[64] Compared with women with postpartum onset of major depression, women who have onset of major depression during pregnancy are more likely to have a prior history of depression and history of typical risk factors for depression, including abuse and low social support.[65,66] Findings from a hormonal challenge study conducted in healthy parturient women with no history of postnatal depression and a comparison group with a history of postpartum depression suggests that both during exposure to and after withdrawal from pregnancy-levels of estradiol and progesterone, women with a history of postpartum depression are vulnerable to develop depression.[5]

There is a remarkable increased risk of mania and psychosis during the first few weeks postpartum, with an incidence of 2.5 to 5 per 10,000 deliveries. Almost all of these episodes are a first episode or recurrence of bipolar I disorder, with a 23-fold increased risk of the first onset of affective psychosis in the postpartum period.[67,68] However, some women may experience these episodes only postpartum and are not otherwise at risk of recurrence.[69] Women with postpartum manic episodes often experience more disorganization, disturbed sensorium, bizarre behavior, and sense of persecution than seen in typical manic episodes.[70,71] Childbirth also seems to be a trigger for hypomanic episodes, which can occur in 10% to 20% of women and in the early postpartum period.[72] Postpartum hypomania may foreshadow the onset of a depression that occurs in about half of women who experience postpartum mood elevation.[68] In addition, women who experience postpartum depression are at increased risk to develop bipolar disorder in long-term follow-up.[73]

OCD symptoms are unusually common in postpartum depression, occurring in up to 35% of women with postpartum onset depression.[65,74] In a survey of adult women with OCD, 32% reported that their OCD symptoms began either during pregnancy or the early postnatal period. Women who reported onset of OCD or worsening of their ongoing OCD symptoms in the perinatal period, were also more likely to indicate that their symptoms worsened premenstrually.[75] Although these findings await confirmation using prospective assessments, they suggest that the hormonal milieu associated with pregnancy, postpartum and the luteal phase of the menstrual cycle may trigger or exacerbate OCD symptoms in a subgroup of hormonally sensitive women. The postpartum period also has been identified as high risk for onset or relapse of panic disorder.[76,77] Finally, there is evidence from a placebo-controlled trial that women are less likely to relapse to cocaine use if treated with progesterone postpartum.[26]

Free thyroxine (T4) levels decrease during pregnancy due to higher levels of thyroid-binding globulin stimulated by increased estrogen levels, enhanced placental and renal clearance of thyroid hormone, increased volume of distribution of thyroid hormone, and suppression of thyroid stimulating hormone.[78] Lower levels of free T4 have been associated with increased depression symptoms in the third trimester of pregnancy.[79,80] In addition, there is preliminary evidence that women with antithyroid antibodies are at increased risk of postpartum onset of depression[81] and postpartum psychosis.[82] An estimated 8% to 15% of reproductive aged women have antithyroid antibodies, most commonly antiperoxidase and antithyroglobulin antibodies.[83] Antibody titers are suppressed during pregnancy, then rebound postpartum. Longitudinal studies estimate a 33% to 50% risk of postpartum thyroiditis in women with antithyroid antibodies, which manifests as hyperthyroidism or hypothyroidism.[84]

LACTATION

Lactating women continue to produce increased amounts of oxytocin and prolactin, which are released into the circulation. It is unclear to what degree increased secretion of these hormones also occurs in the brain but animal studies suggest central activity of these hormones is increased during lactation and that these hormones have anxiolytic effects.[85,86] Compared with postpartum women who are not breast-feeding, lactating women show suppression of the HPA axis and autonomic responses to stress.[87,88] There are also some preliminary reports of reduced rates of depression and anxiety in lactating women, although evidence in contradictory.[89]

MENOPAUSE

Women experience a marked variability of estrogen and progesterone levels in perimenopause. During the menopausal transition, the risk for an episode of major depression is 4-fold to 6-fold greater for women who have a history of major depression and 2-fold to 3-fold for those women with no history of major depression during the childbearing years.[3,90] Prevalence data is sparse for late-life affective disorders but the increased risk for depression in women seems to be lost after menopause.[19] Women do experience an age-independent decline in immediate and delayed verbal recall during the menopausal transition, suggesting that changes in reproductive function affect cognition in addition to mood in some women.[91] In addition, randomized clinical trials[92,93] indicate that typical hormone therapy doses of estradiol (50 or 100 μg/d) are significantly more effective than placebo in treating major depression with perimenopausal onset but not major depression that onsets after menopause.[94]

Several recent placebo-controlled trials have demonstrated a beneficial effect of raloxifene, a selective receptor estrogen modulator on multiple symptom domains of schizophrenia in perimenopausal and postmenopausal women.[95,96] These reports are consistent with observational evidence of a protective effect of female reproductive hormones in schizophrenia. Women have been reported to have a second peak of schizophrenia onset at age 45 to 49 years[97] and to be at higher risk for schizophrenia between 50 and 70 years.[98] There is also evidence for a decline in antipsychotic response for women with schizophrenia after menopause, with increasing duration of menopause and with less lifetime estrogen exposure.[99,100] Progesterone may also affect the course of schizophrenia, in part due to modulation of dopaminergic systems; however, this possibility has not been studied in clinical trials.[101]

SUMMARY

Puberty, the menstrual cycle, pregnancy, and menopause are clearly triggers for onset, recurrence, and exacerbation of affective and anxiety disorders in some women. There is also evidence for estrogen modulation of schizophrenia symptoms. Mood and anxiety disorders are highly comorbid and have shared symptoms and familial risk,[102–104] suggesting that some of the same mechanisms are likely contributing to increased female vulnerability and sensitivity to gonadal steroid changes across this group of disorders. Evidence for effects of postpubertal reproductive events or exogenous hormone treatments on other psychiatric disorders is not strong. Hormonal effects during development may contribute to sex differences in the prevalence of other psychiatric disorders, such as autism and tic disorders, but chromosomal sex differences could also play a role. At this point, the brain systems and biological mechanisms mediating the psychiatric effects of hormonal fluxes in women are not well understood. The hormonal milieu is quite different in the vulnerable periods of the luteal phase, postpartum, and perimenopause. There are little longitudinal data to determine whether the same or different women are most vulnerable to mood dysregulation during these distinct reproductive events that involve changes in multiple hormones and hormone metabolites, and multiple downstream brain systems.

REFERENCES

1. Epperson C, Steiner M, Hartlage S, et al. Premenstrual dysphoric disorder: evidence for a new category for DSM-5. Am J Psychiatry 2012;169:465–75.
2. Gaynes B, Gavin N, Meltzer-Brody S, et al. Perinatal depression: prevalence, screening accuracy, and screening outcomes. Evid Rep Technol Assess vol. 119. Rockville (MD): AHRQ Publication No. 05-E006-s; 2005. p. 1–8.
3. Freeman E, Sammel M, Boorman D, et al. Longitudinal pattern of depressive symptoms around natural menopause. JAMA Psychiatry 2014;71:36–43.
4. Schmidt PJ, Nieman LK, Danaceau MA, et al. Differential behavioral effects of gonadal steroids in women with and in those without premenstrual syndrome. N Engl J Med 1998;338:209–16.
5. Bloch M, Scmidt PJ, Danaceau M, et al. Effects of gonadal steroids in women with a history of postpartum depression. Am J Psychiatry 2000;157:924–30.
6. Curley J, Jensen C, Mashoodh R, et al. Social influences on neurobiology and behavior: epigenetic effects during development. Psychoneuroendocrinology 2011;36:352–71.
7. Kessler R, McGonagle K, Zhao S, et al. Lifetime and 12-month prevalence of DSM-III-R psychiatric disorders in the United States. Results from the National Comorbidity Survey. Arch Gen Psychiatry 1994;51:8–19.
8. Kessler R, Sonnega A, Bromet E, et al. Posttraumatic stress disorder in the National Comorbidity Survey. Arch Gen Psychiatry 1995;52:1048–60.
9. Gater R, Tansella M, Korten A, et al. Sex differences in the prevalence and detection of depressive and anxiety disorders in general health care settings: report from the World Health Organization Collaborative Study on Psychological Problems in General Health Care. Arch Gen Psychiatry 1998;55:405–13.
10. Weissman M, Bland R, Canino G, et al. The cross national epidemiology of obsessive compulsive disorder. The Cross National Collaborative Group. J Clin Psychiatry 1994;55(Suppl):5–10.
11. Liebenluft E. Women with bipolar disorder: an update. Bull Menninger Clin 2000; 64:5–13.
12. Kessler R, Rubinow D, Holmes C. The epidemiology of DSM-III-R bipolar I disorder in a general population survey. Psychol Med 1997;27:1079–89.
13. Angst J. The course of affective disorders, II: typology of bipolar manic-depressive illness. Arch Psych Neurol Sci 1978;226:65–73.

14. Hankin B. Development of sex differences in depressive and co-occurring anxious symptoms during adolescence: descriptive trajectories and potential explanations in a multiwave prospective study. J Clin Child Adolesc Psychol 2009;38:460–72.
15. Nolen-Hoeksema S, Larson J, Grayson C. Explaining the gender difference in depressive symptoms. J Pers Soc Psychol 1999;77:1061–72.
16. Arnold A. The organizational-activational hypothesis as the foundation for a unified theory of sexual differentiation of all mammalian tissues. Horm Behav 2009; 55:570–8.
17. McCarthy M, Arnold A, Ball G, et al. Sex differences in the brain: The not so inconvenient truth. J Neurosci 2012;32:2241–7.
18. Finegan J, Bartleman B, Wong P. A window for the study of prenatal sex hormone influences on postnatal development. J Genet Psychol 1989;150:101–12.
19. Quigley C. Editorial: the postnatal gonadotropin and sex steroid surge-insights from the androgen insensitivity syndrome. J Clin Endocrinol Metab 2002;87: 24–8.
20. DeZegher F, Devlieger H, Veldhuis J. Pulsatile and sexually dimorphic secretion of luteinizing hormone in the human infant on the day of birth. Pediatr Res 1992; 32:605–7.
21. Lombardo M, Ashwin E, Auyeung B, et al. Fetal programming effects of testosterone on the reward system and behavioral approach tendencies in humans. Biol Psychiatry 2012;72:839–47.
22. Arnold AP, Chen X, Itoh Y. What a difference an X or Y makes: sex chromosomes, gene dose, and epigenetics in sexual differentiation. Handb Exp Pharmacol 2012;(214):67–88.
23. Seney M, Ekong K, Ding Y, et al. Sex chromosome complement regulates expression of mood-related genes. Biol Sex Differ 2013;4:20.
24. Raznahan A, Probst F, Palmert M, et al. High resolution whole brain imaging of anatomical variation in XO, XX, and XY mice. Neuroimage 2013;83:962–8.
25. Lee J, Harley V. The male flight-fright response: a result of SRY regulation of catecholamines? Bioessays 2012;34:454–7.
26. Dietz D, Laplant Q, Watts E, et al. Paternal transmission of stress-induced pathologies. Biol Psychiatry 2011;70:408–14.
27. Zaidan H, Leshem M, Gaisler-Salomon I. Prereproductive stress to female rats alters corticotropin releasing factor type 1 expression in ova and behavior and brain corticotropin releasing factor type 1 expression in offspring. Biol Psychiatry 2013;74:680–7.
28. Sandman C, Glynn L, Davis E. Is there a viability-vulnerability tradeoff? Sex differences in fetal programming. J Psychosom Res 2013;75:327–35.
29. Buss C, Davis E, Shahbaba B, et al. Maternal cortisol over the course of pregnancy and subsequent child amygdala and hippocampus volumes and affective problems. Proc Natl Acad Sci U S A 2012;109:1312–9.
30. Grey K, Davis E, Sandman C, et al. Human milk cortisol is associated with infant temperment. Psychoneuroendocrinology 2012;38:1178–85.
31. Lewinsohn P, Gotlieb I, Lewinsohn M, et al. Gender differences in anxiety disorders and anxiety symptoms in adolescents. J Abnorm Psychol 1998;107: 109–17.
32. Nolen-Hoeksema S, Girgus J. The emergence of gender differences in depression during adolescence. Psychol Bull 1994;115:424–43.
33. Angold A, Costello E, Worthman C. Puberty and depression: the roles of age, pubertal status and pubertal timing. Psychol Med 1998;28:51–61.

34. Patton G, Coffey C, Carlin J, et al. Prematurity at birth and adolescent depression. Br J Psychiatry 2004;184:446–7.
35. Costello E, Worthman C, Erkanli A, et al. Predicting from low birth weight to female adolescent depression. A test of competing hypotheses. Arch Gen Psychiatry 2007;64:338–44.
36. van Lieshout R, Boylan K. Increased depressive symptoms in female but not male adolescents born at low birth weight in the offspring of a national cohort. Can J Psychiatry 2010;55:422–9.
37. Rice F, Jones I, Thapar A. The impact of gestational stress and prenatal growth on emotional problems in offspring: a review. Acta Psychiatr Scand 2007;115: 171–83.
38. Ge X, Lorenz F, Conger R, et al. Trajectories of stressful life events and depressive symptoms during adolescence. Dev Psychol 1994;30:467–83.
39. Hankin B, Mermelstein R, Roesch L. Sex differences in adolescent depression: Stress exposure and reactivity models. Child Dev 2007;78:279–95.
40. Copeland W, Angold A, Shanahan L, et al. Longitudinal Patterns of Anxiety From Childhood to Adulthood: The Great Smoky Mountains Study. J Am Acad Child Adolesc Psychiatry 2014;53:21–33.
41. Haley C, Sung S, Rush A, et al. The clinical relevance of self-reported premenstrual worsening of depressive symptoms in the management of depressed outpatients: a STAR*D report. J Womens Health 2013;22:219–29.
42. Rubinow D, Hoban M, Grover G, et al. Changes in plasma hormones across the menstrual cycle in patients with menstrually related mood disorder and in control subjects. Am J Obstet Gynecol 1988;158:5–11.
43. Schmidt P, Nieman L, Grover G, et al. Lack of effect of induced menses on symptoms in women with premenstrual syndrome. N Engl J Med 1991;324: 1174–9.
44. Pinna G, Costa E, Guidotti A. SSRIs act as selective brain steroidoenic stimulants (SBSSs) at low doses that are inactive on 5-HT reuptake. Curr Opin Pharmacol 2009;9:24–30.
45. Uzunov D, Cooper T, Costa E, et al. Fluoxetine-elicited changes in brain neurosteroid content measured by negative ion mass fragmentography. Proc Natl Acad Sci U S A 1996;93:12599–604.
46. Porcu P, O'Buckley T, Alward S, et al. Simultaneous quantification of GABAergic 3alpha,5alpha/3alpha,5ß neuroactive steroids in human and rat serum. Steroids 2009;74:463–73.
47. Yonkers K, Altemus M, Cameron B, et al. The influence of cyclic hormonal contraception on expression of premenstrual syndrome. J Womens Health 2016. [Epub ahead of print].
48. Kim D, Czarkowski K, Epperson C. The relationship between bipolar disorder, seasonality, and premenstrual symptoms. Curr Psychiatry Rep 2011;13:500–3.
49. Teatro M, Mazmanian D, Sharma V. Effects of the menstrual cycle on bipolar disorder. Bipolar Disord 2014;16:22–36.
50. van Veen J, Jonker B, van Vliet I, et al. The effects of female reproductive hormones in generalized social anxiety disorder. Int J Psychiatry Med 2009;39: 283–95.
51. Klump K, Keel P, Racine S, et al. he interactive effects of estrogen and progesterone on changes in emotional eating across the menstrual cycle. J Abnorm Psychol 2013;122:131–7.

52. Soni M, Curran V, Kamboj S. Identification of a narrow post-ovulatory window of vulnerability to distressing involuntary memories in healthy women. Neurobiol Learn Mem 2013;104:32–8.
53. Bergemann N, Parzer P, Nagl I, et al. Acute psychiatric admission and menstrual cycle phase in women withschizophrenia. Arch Womens Ment Health 2002;5: 119–26.
54. Rubin L, Carter C, Drogos L, et al. Peripheral oxytocin is associated with reduced symptom severity in schizophrenia. Schizophr Res 2010;124:13–21.
55. Bergemann N, Parzer P, Runnebaum B, et al. Estrogen, menstrual cycle phases, and psychopathology in women suffering from schizophrenia. Psychol Med 2007;37:1427–36.
56. Panagiotakopoulos L, Neigh G. Development of the HPA axis: where and when do sex differences manifest? Front Neuroendocrinol 2014;35(3):285–302.
57. Kudielka B, Kirschbaum C. Sex differences in HPA axis responses to stress: a review. Psychoneuroendocrinology 2005;69:113–32.
58. Altemus M, Redwine L, Leong YM, et al. Reduced sensitivity to glucocorticoid feedback and reduced glucocorticoid receptor mRNA expression in the luteal phase of the menstrual cycle. Neuropsychopharmacology 1997;17:100–9.
59. Roca C, Schmidt P, Altemus M, et al. Differential menstrual cycle regulation of hypothalamic-pituitary-adrenal axis in women with premenstrual syndrome and controls. J Clin Endocrinol Metab 2003;88:3057–63.
60. Kirschbaum C, Kudielka B, Gaab J, et al. Impact of gender, menstrual cycle phase, and oral contraceptive on the activity of the hypothalamic-pituitary-adrenal axis. Psychosom Med 1999;61:154–62.
61. Altemus M, Fong J, Yang R, et al. Changes in CSF neurochemistry during pregnancy. Biol Psychiatry 2004;56:386–92.
62. Zaconeta A, Amato A, Barra G, et al. Cerebrospinal fluid CRH levels in late pregnancy are not associated with new-onset postpartum depressive symptoms. J Clin Endocrinol Metab 2015;100:3159–64.
63. AmericanPsychiatricAssociation. Diagnostic and statistical manual of mental disorders, 5th edition (DSM-5). Washington, DC: American Psychiatric Publishing; 2013.
64. Wisner K, Sit D, McShea M, et al. Onset timing, thoughts of self-harm, and diagnoses in postpartum women with screen-positive depression findings. JAMA Psychiatry 2013;70:490–8.
65. Altemus M, Neeb C, Davis A, et al. Phenotypic differences between pregnancy-onset and postpartum-onset major depressive disorder. J Clin Psychiatry 2013; 73:e1485–1491.
66. Stowe Z, Hostetter A, Newport D. The onset of postpartum depression: Implications for clinical screening in obstetrical and primary care. Am J Obstet Gynecol 2005;192:522–6.
67. Munk-Olsen T, Laursen T, Pedersen C, et al. New parents and mental disorders. JAMA 2006;296:2582–9.
68. Sharma V, Pope C. Pregnancy and bipolar disorder: a systematic review. J Clin Psychiatry 2012;73:1447–55.
69. Chaudron L, Pies R. The relationship between postpartum psychosis and bipolar disorder: a review. J Clin Psychiatry 2003;64:1284–92.
70. Wisner K, Peindl K, Hanusa B. Symptomatology of affective and psychotic illnesses related to childbearing. J Affect Disord 1994;30:77–87.
71. Brockington I, Cernik A, Schfield E, et al. Puerperal psychosis, phenomena and diagnosis. Arch Gen Psychiatry 1981;38:829–33.

72. Heron J, Haque S, Oyebode F, et al. A longitudinal study of hypomania and depression symptoms in pregnancy and the postpartum period. Bipolar Disord 2009;11:410–7.
73. Munk-Olsen T, Laursen T, Meltzer-Brody S, et al. Psychiatric disorders with postpartum onset: possible early manifestations of bipolar affective disorders. Arch Gen Psychiatry 2012;69:428–34.
74. Wisner K, Peindl K, Gigliotti T, et al. Obsessions and compulsions in women with postpartum depression. J Clin Psychiatry 1999;60:176–80.
75. Forray A, Focseneanu M, Pittman B, et al. Onset and exacerbation of obsessive-compulsive disorder in pregnancy and the postpartum period. J Clin Psychiatry 2010;71(8):1061–8.
76. Sholomskas DE, Wickamaratne PJ, Dogolo L, et al. Postpartum onset of panic disorder: a coincidental event? J Clin Psychiatry 1993;54:476–80.
77. Klein D. Pregnancy and panic disorder. J Clin Psychiatry 1994;55:293–4.
78. Glinoer D. The regulation of thyroid function in pregnancy: pathways of endocrine adaptation from physiology to pathology. Endocr Rev 1997;18:404–43.
79. Pedersen C, Johnson J, Silva S, et al. Antenatal thyroid correlates of postpartum depression. Psychoneuroendocrinology 2007;32:235–45.
80. Pedersen C, Stern R, Pate J, et al. Thyroid and adrenal measures during late pregnancy and the puerperium in women who have been major depressed or who become dysphoric postpartum. J Affect Disord 1993;29:201–11.
81. Kuijpens J, Vader H, Drexhage H, et al. Thyroid peroxidase antibodies during gestation are a marker for subsequent depression postpartum. Eur J Endocrinol 2001;145:579–84.
82. Bergink V, Kushner S, Pop V, et al. Prevalence of autoimmune thyroid dysfunction in postpartum psychosis. Br J Psychiatry 2011;198:264–8.
83. Watson J, Mednick S, Huttunen M, et al. Prenatal teratogens and the development of adult mental illness. Dev Psychopathol 1999;11:457–66.
84. Nicholson W, Robinson K, Smallridge R, et al. Prevalence of postpartum thyroid dysfunction: a quantitative review. Thyroid 2006;16:573–82.
85. Neumann ID, Torner L, Wigger A. Brain oxytocin: differential inhibition of neuroendocrine stress responses and anxiety-related behaviour in virgin, pregnant and lactating rats. Neuroscience 2000;95:567–75.
86. Torner L, Toschi N, Pohlinger A, et al. Anxioolytic and anti-stress effects of brain prolactin: improved antisense efficacy of antisense targeting of the prolactin receptor by molecular modeling. J Neurosci 2001;21:3207–14.
87. Altemus M, Deuster P, Galliven E, et al. Suppression of hypothalamic-pituitary-adrenal axis responses to stress in lactating women. J Clin Endocrinol Metab 1995;80:2954–9.
88. Altemus M, Redwine LS, Leong Y-M, et al. Responses to laboratory psychosocial stress in postpartum women. Psychosom Med 2001;63:814–21.
89. Pope C, Maxmanian D. Breastfeeding and postpartum depression: an overview and methodological recommendations for future research. Depress Res Treat 2016;2016:4765310.
90. Cohen L, Soares C, Vitonis A, et al. Risk for new onset of depression during the menopausal transition: the Harvard Study of Moods and Cycles. Arch Gen Psychiatry 2006;63:375–82.
91. Epperson C, Sammel M, Freeman E. Menopause effects on verbal memory: findings from a longitudinal community cohort. J Clin Endocrinol Metab 2013;98:3829–38.

92. Schmidt P, Nieman L, Danaceau M, et al. Estrogen replacement in perimenopause-related depression: a preliminary report. Am J Obstet Gynecol 2000;183:414–20.
93. Soares C, Almeida O, Joffe H, et al. Efficacy of estradiol for the treatment of depressive disorders in perimenopausal women: a double-blind, randomized, placebo-controlled trial. Arch Gen Psychiatry 2001;58:529–34.
94. Morrison M, Kallan M, Have T, et al. Lack of efficacy of estradiol for depression in postmenopausal women: a randomized, controlled trial. Biol Psychiatry 2004; 55:406–12.
95. Usall J, Huerta-Ramos E, Labad J, et al. Raloxifene as an Adjunctive Treatment for Postmenopausal Women With Schizophrenia: A 24-Week Double-Blind, Randomized, Parallel, Placebo-Controlled Trial. Schizophr Bull 2016;42:309–17.
96. Kulkarni J, Gavrilidis E, Gwini S, et al. Effect of Adjunctive Raloxifene Therapy on Severity of Refractory Schizophrenia in Women: A Randomized Clinical Trial. JAMA Psychiatry 2016;73:947–54.
97. Hafner H. Gender differences in schizophrenia. Psychoneuroendocrinology 2003;28:17–54.
98. van derWerf M, Hanssen M, Kohler S, et al. Systematic review and collaborative recalculation of 133,693 incident cases of schizophrenia. Psychol Med 2014;44:9–16.
99. González-Rodríguez A, Catalán R, Penadés R, et al. Antipsychotic response worsens with postmenopausal duration in women with schizophrenia. J Clin Psychopharmacol 2016;36:580–7.
100. Goldstein J, Cohen L, Horton N. Sex differences in clinical response to olanzapine compared with haloperidol. Psychiatry Res 2002;110:27–37.
101. Sun J, Walker A, Dean B, et al. Progesterone: The neglected hormone in schizophrenia? A focus on progesterone-dopamine interactions. Psychoneuroendocrinology 2016;74:126–40.
102. Kotov R, Ruggero C, Krueger R, et al. New dimensions in the quantitative classification of mental illness. Arch Gen Psychiatry 2011;68:1003–11.
103. Angold A, Costello E, Erkanli A. Comorbidity. J Child Psychol Psychiatry 1999; 40:57–87.
104. Kravitz H, Schott L, Joffe H, et al. Do anxiety symptoms predict major depressive disorder in midlife women? The Study of Women's Health Across the Nation (SWAN) Mental Health Study (MHS). Psychol Med 2014;44(12):2593–602.

Premenstrual Dysphoric Disorder

Teresa Lanza di Scalea, MD, PhD[a,*], Teri Pearlstein, MD[b]

KEYWORDS

- Premenstrual syndrome • Premenstrual dysphoric disorder • Etiology
- Antidepressant • Oral contraceptive • Treatment

KEY POINTS

- Premenstrual dysphoric disorder comprises psychological and somatic symptoms and functional impairment that lie on the severe end of the continuum of premenstrual symptoms.
- Etiologic theories include differential response to normal hormonal fluctuations that may involve the serotonin system, the neurosteroid allopregnanalone, or luteal phase changes in brain circuitry involving emotional and cognitive function.
- Serotonin reuptake inhibitors are considered the first-line treatment option and may be taken continuously, for the full premenstrual phase or as "symptom-onset" dosing.
- Second-line treatments include oral contraceptives containing drospirenone, other ovulation suppression methods, calcium, chasteberry, and cognitive-behavioral therapy.

DEFINITION

Premenstrual psychological and somatic symptoms lie on a continuum of severity. It is estimated that about 85% of women experience at least one mild premenstrual symptom; 20% to 25% experience moderate to severe premenstrual symptoms (premenstrual syndrome or PMS), and about 5% meet diagnostic criteria for premenstrual dysphoric disorder (PMDD),[1] the severest form of PMS.

Currently, the most liberal diagnostic criteria is found in International Statistical Classification of Diseases and Related Health Problems, 10th revision, from the World Health Organization, in which "Premenstrual Tension Syndrome" is met if at least one

This article originally appeared in the *Psychiatric Clinics of North America*, Volume 40, Issue 2, June 2017.
Disclosures: Neither author has any commercial or financial conflicts of interest or any funding source for this article.
[a] Assistant Professor of Psychiatry and Women's Health, Dell Medical School, University of Texas at Austin, Austin, TX, USA; [b] Department of Psychiatry and Human Behavior, Alpert Medical School of Brown University, Women's Behavioral Medicine, Women's Medicine Collaborative, Miriam Hospital, 146 West River Street, Providence, RI 02904, USA
* Corresponding author.
E-mail address: teresa.lanza@austin.utexas.edu

Med Clin N Am 103 (2019) 613–628
http://dx.doi.org/10.1016/j.mcna.2019.02.007 medical.theclinics.com

premenstrual symptom is present, without specification of severity and with no requirement of prospective ratings. The criteria from the American College of Obstetrics and Gynecology and the Royal College of Obstetricians and Gynecologists describe PMS as any number of psychological or physical symptoms; however, functional impairment is required and prospective ratings are recommended.[2] The International Society for Premenstrual Disorders defines Core Premenstrual Disorder as psychological and/or somatic symptoms that occur in the luteal phase of ovulatory cycles; the symptoms should cause functional impairment and be prospectively rated over 2 menstrual cycles.[2]

The American Psychiatric Association publishes the PMDD diagnostic criteria in the Diagnostic and Statistical Manual of Mental Disorders (DSM).[1] Symptoms must be present during the last week before the onset of menstruation, start to improve within a few days from the onset of menses, should be minimal or absent in the weeks after menses, and should be present most cycles of the past year. A minimum of 5 symptoms must be present, including one "core" symptom (marked affective lability, irritability, depressed mood, or anxiety) with other potential symptoms that include decreased interest in usual activities, difficulty concentrating, low energy, changes in sleep or appetite, sense of being overwhelmed or out of control, and physical symptoms. The premenstrual symptoms should be associated with significant distress or interference in functioning. The premenstrual symptoms should not be merely an exacerbation of the symptoms of another psychiatric disorder and should not be attributable to the effects of a medication, substance, or medical condition. The timing of the symptoms should be confirmed by prospective daily ratings for 2 menstrual cycles, and until prospective ratings are completed, the PMDD diagnosis should be considered "provisional."[1]

In prior editions of the DSM, PMDD was included in the Appendix because it was considered a condition for which additional research was needed before being confirmed as a psychiatric disorder. In the recent DSM-5 edition, PMDD was included for the first time in the main text, categorized as a depressive disorder.[1] This decision was based on evidence showing its distinctiveness from other disorders, specific antecedent validators, concurrent validators, and predictive response to treatment.[3] The change of status of PMDD in the DSM-5 has continued debates about potential negative consequences for women meeting criteria for the disorder.[4–6]

DIAGNOSTIC TOOLS

Rating scales of premenstrual symptoms include visual analogue scales and Likert scale rating forms, the most common of which is the Daily Record of Severity of Problems, in which women rate symptom severity and functional items daily.[7] Prospective ratings confirm the timing of the symptoms and rule out underlying psychiatric disorders that are premenstrually exacerbated. Prospective ratings are time consuming for women to complete and for clinicians to view and score. Steiner and colleagues[8,9] developed a self-report questionnaire, the Premenstrual Symptoms Screening Tool (PSST), which retrospectively assesses premenstrual symptoms and functional impairment over the last menstrual cycle. The PSST is available as adult and adolescent versions. A medical and gynecologic history, a physical examination, and an assessment for thyroid disorders and anemia are suggested as part of the initial evaluation before initiation of treatment.[10,11]

EPIDEMIOLOGY

Using prospective daily ratings, the estimated prevalence of PMDD in adults is 5% and of severe PMS is 20%. Prevalence figures of PMDD in adolescents may be somewhat higher.[9,11] Adult prevalence figures have been consistent across several continents and ethnic populations. In some populations, irritability is the most common symptom, whereas physical symptoms are most common in other populations.[12]

It is not clear if premenstrual symptoms change with age. A prospective study of nearly 1500 adolescents and young adults reported no change in PMDD (not prospectively confirmed) prevalence over a 2-year period.[13] In contrast, in a 10-year prospective evaluation of a nonclinical population, premenstrual symptoms increased from age 21 until age 30.[14] PMDD leads to significant functional impairment and diminished quality of life, comparable to major depressive disorder (MDD) and dysthymia,[15,16] and it is considered responsible for 14.5 million disability adjusted life-years in the United States.[15]

CLINICAL FEATURES

PMDD is associated with depressive and anxiety disorders, both concurrently and in the past. Comorbidity rates between PMDD and other psychiatric disorders were high in a 2-year prospective study of adolescents and young adults; both the 2-year and the lifetime prevalence were the highest for anxiety disorders (47.4%), followed by mood disorders (29.8%).[13] A recent study assessed the lifetime prevalence of psychiatric disorders by structured interview in a sample of women with prospectively confirmed PMDD.[17] Although 45% did not meet criteria for any previous diagnosis, 31.2% met criteria for MDD, 15.3% met criteria for an anxiety disorder, the most frequent of which was panic disorder (6%), and 18.6% met criteria for a substance use disorder.[17] These data are in line with older studies reporting that MDD is the most prevalent lifetime psychiatric disorder in women with PMDD.

Cross-sectional studies have suggested a link between trauma exposure and PMS/PMDD. Participants of an epidemiology survey with a history of trauma or meeting criteria for PTSD were reported to be more likely to have PMDD compared with women with no trauma history.[18] A community-based longitudinal study of adolescents and young adults estimated that previous trauma exposure significantly increased the risk of PMDD onset at 42 months follow-up (odds ratio [OR] 4.2).[19]

Personality disorders do not appear to be significantly elevated in women with PMDD compared with healthy controls, although the literature is mixed. A recent study reported that obsessive compulsive personality disorder was the most prevalent personality disorder in women with severe PMS.[20] Several studies suggest that personality traits may be elevated in women with PMS/PMDD. One study reported that several personality traits were more frequent in women with PMDD compared with healthy controls, and 5 of the traits were significantly associated with polymorphic variants in the estrogen receptor alpha (ESR-1) gene.[21]

Traits of impulsivity, anger, affect intensity, and lability were significantly associated with PMS and PMDD in a recent study of women hospitalized after a suicide attempt.[22] A study of 2400 adolescents and young adults reported that PMS was associated with suicidal attempts.[13] PMDD was reported to be associated with suicidal ideation in 2500 Korean women after adjustment for other psychiatric disorders.[23] In a survey of almost 4000 US women, those with moderate to severe PMS were more likely to endorse suicidal ideation compared with women with no PMS, and women with PMDD were more likely to report 3 suicidality factors (ideation, plans, and attempts) compared with women with no PMDD.[24]

Studies on PMDD being a risk factor for postpartum depression (PPD) have led to mixed results. In postpartum women, a past history of moderate to severe PMS or PMDD (using the PSST) increased the risk of PPD (OR 1.97), whereas a history of depression did not.[25] However, a recent study of 215 women with prospectively confirmed PMDD reported that only a minority of women with PMDD had a history of PPD (7.4%), but nearly 36% had previous MDD.[17] Longitudinal population-based studies reported that retrospectively endorsed PMS is an independent risk factor for depressive symptoms during the menopausal transition.[26,27] A small study reported that perimenopausal women with depression had a higher prevalence of premenstrual dysphoria compared with nondepressed women.[28] Although prospective longitudinal studies are needed, women with PMDD may be at risk for depressive symptoms or MDD during the postpartum period and the menopausal transition due to shared vulnerability to hormonal fluctuations at these time periods.

ETIOLOGIC THEORIES

Etiology theories are summarized in **Box 1**. A seminal study about PMDD cause was conducted by Schmidt and colleagues.[29] Women prospectively diagnosed with PMS and women with no PMS received leuprolide, a gonadotropin-releasing hormone agonist, to achieve ovarian suppression. Subjects continued to receive leuprolide and then received in random order 17-beta-estradiol or progesterone. When estradiol or progesterone was added, women with PMS experienced reappearance of mood and anxiety symptoms, whereas women without PMS did not, indicating that premenstrual symptoms occur due to abnormal response to otherwise physiologic gonadal hormone levels.[29] Multiple other studies have reported that serum concentrations of gonadal hormones do not differ between women with PMDD and women without PMDD. Why the abnormal response occurs in a subset of women, and what constitutes this vulnerability, are not yet fully answered questions.

Recent growing interest focuses on the neurosteroid allopregnanolone (3α, 5α-tetrahydroprogesterone) and its effect on the gamma-aminobutyric acid (GABA) system, one of the main inhibitory systems in the central nervous system. Allopregnanolone is a metabolite of progesterone implicated in mood disorders in both men and women.[30,31] Synthesis first involves the enzymatic conversion of progesterone to 5α-dihydroprogesterone (5α-DHP) by the enzyme 5α-reductase, which is then

Box 1
Etiologic theories of premenstrual dysphoric disorder

1. Abnormal response to normal fluctuations of the hypothalamic-pituitary-gonadal axis
2. Decreased or paradoxic sensitivity of the $GABA_A$ receptor to allopregnanolone
3. Alterations in serotonin system function
4. Alterations in hypothalamic-pituitary-adrenal axis response
5. Altered immune function
6. Altered calcium homeostasis
7. Altered circadian rhythms
8. Genetic factors (eg, polymorphisms in the gene for the ESR1)
9. Abnormal responses in brain regions to emotion processing and regulation during luteal phase

converted to allopregnanolone by the enzyme 3α-hydroxysteroid dehydrogenase (3α-HSD).[30,31] Allopregnanolone is a strong positive modulator of $GABA_A$ receptor, acting on a specific site of the receptor distinct from the site acted on by barbiturates, benzodiazepines, and alcohol, yet similarly to them, leading to increased receptor activity. Preclinical studies suggest that allopregnanolone mediates its own fluctuations as well as the fluctuations of progesterone, through modulation of subunits of $GABA_A$ receptor and receptor function.[32]

It is currently proposed that women with PMDD have reduced sensitivity at the $GABA_A$ receptor complex, at the allopregnanolone, as well as at the benzodiazepine site. Studies using saccadic eye velocity (SEV) (an objective involuntary measure of the sedative/anxiolytic effect of the $GABA_A$ receptor activation in response to benzodiazepines) have shown reduced sensitivity at the $GABA_A$ receptor in PMDD. A recent investigation reported reduced SEV during the follicular phase in women with PMDD who were administered allopregnanolone.[33] Another recent study reported that isoallopregnanolone (an allopregnanolone antagonist) decreased the effect of allopregnanolone on SEV in women with PMDD, confirming the specific effect of allopregnanolone on the $GABA_A$ receptor.[34]

A blunted response to stress has been reported in PMDD, and it has been proposed that a decrease in the expected increase in allopregnanolone in response to stress or reduced allopregnanalone-modulated $GABA_A$ receptor sensitivity impairs the ability of the hypothalamic-pituitary-adrenal axis to achieve homeostasis after stress.[35] Dysregulated acoustic startle responses in women with PMDD suggest increased arousal in the luteal phase, which could be another reflection of dysregulated allopregnanolone function.[36]

In an important recent randomized controlled trial (RCT), when the conversion of progesterone to allopregnanolone was blocked by dutasteride (a 5α-reductase inhibitor), PMDD symptoms were significantly decreased, and there was no effect of dutasteride on the healthy controls.[37] There is a hypothesis that the negative mood and anxiety symptoms of PMDD may be related to a paradoxic sensitivity to allopregnanolone. In a subset of women, when allopregnanolone levels increase (ie, in the midluteal phase), the increase leads to elevated rather than decreased mood and anxiety symptoms.[38,39]

The role of serotonin in the cause of PMS/PMDD is supported by numerous findings using indirect measures of central serotonin and its transmission and by probes of the serotonin system.[40,41] Studies include reduced whole blood serotonin concentration during the luteal phase, reduced serotonin and imipramine binding at the platelet plasma membrane serotonin transporter, exacerbation of premenstrual irritability and anxiety after tryptophan depletion, delayed plasma prolactin response to fenfluramine, and blunted plasma cortisol and ACTH responses to the serotonergic agent m-chlorophenylpiperazine.[40,41] Fluctuations in estradiol may modulate the serotonin transporter and other aspects of serotonin function as well as brain-derived neurotrophic factor (BDNF).[36] BDNF abnormalities in PMS/PMDD have been mixed.[36,42]

The numerous studies demonstrating the efficacy of serotonergic antidepressants[43] support the role of serotonin in PMDD. The rapid onset of action of selective serotonin reuptake inhibitor (SSRIs) suggests a mechanism of action different than serotonin reuptake inhibition. It has been shown that SSRIs increase the level of central allopregnanolone in both rats and humans.[44] Although the mechanism by which this occurs is not known, it has been proposed that it could involve a direct stimulation of 3α-HSD, the enzyme that catalyzes the reduction of 5α-DHP into allopregnanolone.[45]

The potential contribution of a genetic susceptibility has been investigated for PMDD. Population-based twin studies have estimated that the specific heritability of premenstrual symptoms ranges from 30% to 80%.[3,46] A significant study examined the ESR1 gene as a potential contributor to the genetic susceptibility to PMDD.[47] In this study, 4 single nucleotide polymorphisms in the noncoding protein regions (intron) on the gene for the ESR1 were associated with PMDD. Variations in the intron section of a gene may have significant impact in regulating gene expression, and it has been speculated that ESR1 polymorphism may contribute to altered estrogen receptor signaling and altered sensitivity to otherwise physiologic gonadal hormonal levels.[47] Studies of polymorphism in the serotonin transporter gene and genes of enzymes involved in the synthesis and inactivation of serotonin have led to mostly negative results.[48]

Imaging studies have reported negative bias during the luteal phase to a facial emotion recognition task,[49] increased amygdala response to negative versus neutral stimuli, and decreased top-down emotional regulation by the prefrontal cortex in the luteal phase,[50] as well as greater prefrontal activation in women with PMDD (correlating to symptom severity) compared with healthy controls.[51] Overall, studies suggest increased amygdala responses to negative stimuli and blunted top-down inhibition by the dorsolateral prefrontal cortex in the luteal phase in women with PMDD. Neuroimaging studies during the menstrual cycle and in women with PMS or PMDD have been recently reviewed.[39,52]

TREATMENT

The treatment goal is to relieve premenstrual affective and somatic symptoms. Factors to be taken into account include severity of symptoms, response to previous treatments, contraception needs, conception plans, and treatment modality preferences.[12] The most systematically studied treatments have been the "correction" of the neurotransmitter or neurosteroid dysregulation with antidepressant medications, or the elimination of hormonal fluctuations by suppressing ovulation. There is a relative paucity of data on other treatments.

ANTIDEPRESSANTS

SSRIs are considered first-line treatment of PMDD.[10] Treatment studies of SSRIs in PMS/PMDD have reported response rates of 60% to 90% to SSRIs compared with approximately 30% to 40% to placebo, depending on response criteria.[41,53] In general, the effective SSRI doses are similar to the doses recommended for MDD, and fluoxetine, sertraline, and paroxetine are US Food and Drug Administration (FDA) approved (**Box 2**). A systematic review of 31 RCTs of SSRIs in 4372 women with prospectively confirmed PMS or PMDD included 20 trials with continuous (daily) dosing of fluoxetine, sertraline, paroxetine, citalopram, and escitalopram and 14 trials with intermittent dosing (SSRI administered daily during the luteal phase only from ovulation to menses).[43] Psychological and somatic symptoms and functioning significantly improved with SSRIs compared with placebo. The efficacy of continuous and intermittent dosing was equivalent. The most common adverse effects with SSRIs, which were dose related, included nausea, decreased energy, somnolence, fatigue, decreased libido, and sweating.[43] A meta-analysis of 29 placebo-controlled RCTs in 2964 women with severe PMS and PMDD also reported efficacy of SSRIs.[54] However, this meta-analysis concluded that continuous dosing regimens were more effective than intermittent regimens.[54] Studies involving intermittent dosing reported the absence of discontinuation symptoms when fluoxetine, sertraline, and paroxetine were abruptly stopped the first day of menses,[41] presumably due to the short exposure not leading to downregulation of postsynaptic receptors. Intermittent dosing

Box 2
Treatments for premenstrual dysphoric disorder

A. Antidepressant medications
- Fluoxetine 20 mg daily[a]
- Sertraline 50 to 150 mg daily[a]
- Paroxetine CR 12.5 to 25 mg daily[a]
- Citalopram 5 to 20 mg daily
- Escitalopram 10 to 20 mg daily
- Venlafaxine 75 mg daily
- Clomipramine 25 to 75 mg daily

B. Ovulation suppression
- Yaz (oral contraceptive containing ethinyl estradiol 20 μg/drospirenone 3 mg)[b]
- Transdermal estrogen
- GnRH agonist (eg, leuprolide 3.75–7.5 mg intramuscularly monthly)
- Danazol 200 to 400 mg daily

C. Other treatments
- Alprazolam 0.25 mg twice a day during luteal phase
- Bromocriptine for mastalgia
- Spironolactone for bloating
- Calcium 600 mg twice a day
- Chasteberry
- Cognitive-behavioral therapy

[a]Approved by the FDA for full cycle and luteal phase dosing.

[b]Approved by the FDA for women desiring contraception.

may be less effective than continuous dosing for premenstrual physical symptoms.[41,55]

Although the mechanism underlying the quick efficacy of SSRIs in PMDD is not fully elucidated, an increase in allopregnanolone or neuromodulation of estrogen may be involved.[56,57] One study confirmed that an SSRI may relieve premenstrual symptoms within 48 hours.[57] A review reported that for some women, "symptom-onset" dosing (ie, administering SSRIs from the postovulatory day that symptoms appear until menses) may be as effective as continuous or luteal phase dosing.[56] A recent RCT evaluated symptom-onset dosing of sertraline 50 to 100 mg daily taken on symptomatic premenstrual days compared with placebo in 252 women with PMDD. Sertraline (taken an average of 6 premenstrual days) was superior to placebo, particularly for irritability and anger.[58] Symptom-onset dosing may have a unique role when women are trying to conceive (to minimize exposure), during the menopausal transition when menses become irregular, and to mitigate long-term side effects of weight gain and sexual dysfunction.

Studies with the serotonin norepinephrine reuptake inhibitors have been fewer. Continuous dosing of venlafaxine was reported to be superior to placebo in one RCT, and open studies of intermittent use of venlafaxine and continuous use of duloxetine suggested benefit.[41,55] The efficacy of lower doses of venlafaxine may be due to its acting as an SSRI at lower doses. RCTs have also reported efficacy with clomipramine, a tricyclic antidepressant with largely serotonergic action, in daily dosing and luteal phase dosing (see **Box 2**).[41] Three early RCTs that compared SSRIs with nonserotonergic antidepressants and placebo each reported efficacy of the SSRI over placebo and the nonserotonergic antidepressant.[41,55] The differential superiority of SSRIs compared with noradrenergic antidepressants is compatible with the presumed serotonin dysfunction in PMDD and is a potent predictive validator of PMDD as a distinct disorder from mood disorders.[3]

The question of differential efficacy of an SSRI for different premenstrual symptom profiles was examined in 476 women who had participated in PMS/PMDD studies with sertraline.[59] Sertraline was superior to placebo for women with prominent psychological symptoms or mixed psychological and physical symptoms. However, sertraline was not effective for women with predominantly physical premenstrual symptoms and not very severe emotional symptoms.[59] A lack of efficacy of SSRIs for premenstrual headaches has been reported in other studies.

Clinically, many women have noted the recurrence of premenstrual symptoms after SSRI discontinuation, and there is no recommended optimal length of treatment. An RCT examined the relapse of PMS/PMDD with long-term use of an SSRI and following its discontinuation.[60] Women who responded to sertraline 50 to 100 mg daily were discontinued after 4 months or 1 year. Relapse occurred in 60% of women after 4 months of treatment (median time to relapse was 4 months) compared with relapse in 41% of women after 1 year of treatment (median time to relapse was 8 months). Relapse was more likely if a woman had more severe symptoms before treatment and if she had not achieved full symptom remission with sertraline before discontinuation.[60]

Systematic studies are needed of the "bumping up," or semi-intermittent dosing (SSRI dose is increased during the luteal phase and decreased to the usual dose at menses) in women with premenstrual exacerbation of an underlying depressive or anxiety disorder.[56] Studies are also needed of combined treatment in women with PMDD, such as SSRI with hormonal treatment or psychosocial treatment. Preliminary positive reports suggest a potential role of addition of an oral contraceptive (OC) to women with premenstrual exacerbation of MDD[61] and with comorbid bipolar disorder and PMDD.[62]

ORAL CONTRACEPTIVES

OCs have been commonly prescribed by clinicians for the treatment of PMS, but until recently there was minimal literature endorsing their efficacy. Recent RCTs have been conducted with OCs containing drosperinone, a progesterone with unique antimineralocorticoid and antiandrogenic properties. A review reported that OCs containing drosperinone were more effective than placebo in decreasing symptoms of PMS and PMDD after 3 months,[63] noting a high placebo response and nausea, intermenstrual bleeding, and breast pain as common side effects. The review concluded that it is unknown if drosperinone-containing OCs work longer than 3 months or are more effective than OCs with other progestogens.[63] Two studies included in the review involved ethinyl estradiol 20 μg and drospirenone 3 mg (Yaz), administered as 24 days of active pills followed by a 4-day hormone-free interval (24/4). In both a 3-month parallel study in 450 women with PMDD[64] and a crossover design study in 64 women with PMDD,[65] Yaz was superior to placebo in reducing premenstrual emotional and physical symptoms and improving quality of life. In 2006, Yaz received FDA approval for the treatment of PMDD in women desiring OC contraception. In 2012, the FDA added a warning about drosperinone-containing OCs being associated with a higher risk of venous thromboembolism than OCs containing the progestin levonorgestrel or other progestins. Although not definitive that drosperinone-containing OCs uniquely elevate this risk, women considering the start of an OC need an individualized risk assessment.[11]

No RCTs have compared drosperinone-containing OCs to OCs containing other progestogens in women with prospectively confirmed PMS or PMDD. A few RCTs have examined the efficacy of continuous OC use, usually administered for 6 cycles. A review of 4 studies of continuous levonorgestrel 90 μg/ethinyl estradiol 20 μg reported inconsistent results and high placebo responses in women with PMDD.[66,67] An RCT in women with PMS (not prospectively confirmed) reported that Yaz was more effective than desogestrel 150 μg/ethinyl estradiol 20 μg for premenstrual mood and anxiety symptoms after 6 cycles.[68] OCs are considered a second-line treatment for PMDD,[10] and the current evidence suggests that the first-choice OC would be drosperinone 3 mg/ethinyl estradiol 20 μg administered in a 24/4 or continuous regimen.[11]

OTHER OVULATION-SUPPRESSION TREATMENTS

Gonadotropin releasing hormone (GnRH) agonists suppress ovulation by downregulating GnRH receptors in the hypothalamus, leading to decreased follicle-stimulating hormone and luteinizing hormone release from the pituitary, resulting in decreased estrogen and progesterone levels (see **Box 2**). A meta-analysis of 5 studies reported an OR of 8.66 that GnRH agonists will lead to improvement in premenstrual emotional and physical symptoms compared with placebo.[69] After relief is achieved with a GnRH agonist, "add-back" hormone strategies have been investigated due to the medical consequences of the hypoestrogenic state resulting from prolonged anovulation. Although in a couple of studies, the "add-back" of estrogen and progesterone to the GnRH agonist was associated with the reappearance of mood and anxiety symptoms, the meta-analysis concluded that "add-back" hormones did not reduce the efficacy of GnRH agonists.[69] Because women with severe PMS and PMDD have an abnormal response to normal hormonal fluctuations,[29] it is not surprising that some women may have the induction of mood and anxiety symptoms from the addition of gonadal steroids, reducing the benefit of the replacement strategy. It has been suggested to use as low dose as possible "add-back" hormones.[12]

Anovulation achieved with the administration of estrogen (gel, patch, or implant) is commonly used in Europe. Most studies have examined transdermal estrogen for PMS,[53,70] which leads to the same long-term health issues as with GnRH agonists. Protection of the uterus from endometrial hyperplasia can be achieved with a cyclical progestogen, tibolone, or a levonorgestrel-releasing intrauterine system.[12,70] Danazol, a synthetic steroid, alleviates premenstrual symptoms when administered at doses that induce anovulation; however, it is rarely used due to its adverse effects.[12,41]

Hysterectomy with bilateral oophorectomy is considered a last-resort treatment option for women with severe PMDD who do not respond to or cannot tolerate more conventional treatments.[12,41] Confirmation of successful alleviation of PMDD by medical suppression of ovulation should precede a surgical treatment for PMDD.[12,41]

OTHER MEDICATIONS

Luteal phase progesterone (given as vaginal suppositories or oral micronized tablets) has mixed results for PMS or PMDD, largely due to methodological shortcomings of previous studies.[71]

Luteal phase alprazolam is superior to placebo for premenstrual emotional symptoms in most but not all studies.[53,55] Alprazolam should be tapered over the first few days of menses each cycle. A single-blind study reported that both full-cycle buspirone 10 mg daily and fluoxetine 20 mg daily reduced premenstrual symptoms,[72] extending earlier positive reports with luteal phase buspirone.[55] Spironolactone has been reported to decrease premenstrual emotional and physical symptoms and bromocriptine to decrease premenstrual breast tenderness.[53] Mood stabilizers have received minimal study; positive case reports with lamotrigine[73] and levetiracetam[74] have been reported. Adjunctive quetiapine was reported to be helpful in SSRI nonresponders in a small RCT.[75]

DIETARY SUPPLEMENTS

An RCT in 466 women with PMDD reported that calcium 600 mg twice daily was superior to placebo for many emotional and physical premenstrual symptoms.[76] Although calcium may be efficacious compared with placebo, it has less effectiveness than fluoxetine[77] or an OC containing drosperinone compared with placebo.[78] Systematic reviews of vitamin B_6 for the treatment of PMS have reported weak superiority compared with placebo.[79,80] Mixed findings have been reported with studies of essential fatty acids, vitamin E, magnesium, and soy isoflavones.[80] Preliminary RCTs have reported success with vitamin D, tryptophan, wheat germ, and fish oil.

HERBAL AND COMPLEMENTARY TREATMENTS

Results of studies of herbal treatments are difficult to interpret due to the lack of standardization of herb preparations.[81] Evidence-based reviews of complementary treatments have reported that the strongest evidence exists for benefit with chasteberry, or *Vitex agnus-castus*.[80,81] A review reported superior efficacy of chasteberry in women with PMS compared with placebo, pyridoxine, or magnesium, and mixed results compared with fluoxetine.[82] It is hypothesized that the benefit of chasteberry for premenstrual symptoms could be due to its being a dopamine agonist with inhibition of prolactin or increase in melatonin secretion.[82] Initial positive RCTs have been reported for lavender, saffron, ginkgo biloba, and hypericum.[80] A recent report suggested that curcumin (from turmeric) was superior to placebo, possibly by increasing BDNF levels.[42]

Both light therapy and sleep deprivation may decrease premenstrual dysphoria by correcting abnormal circadian and biological rhythms of sleep.[83,84] Optimal duration of these treatments and whether the clinical effect is sustained are unclear. A meta-analysis of RCTs of acupuncture suggested some improvement in premenstrual symptoms but many of the studies contained methodological flaws.[85] There have also been initial positive reports of Qi therapy, massage, yoga, reflexology, biofeedback, chiropractic manipulation, guided imagery, photic stimulation, repetitive transmagnetic stimulation, and other homeopathic treatments.

LIFESTYLE MODIFICATIONS AND PSYCHOSOCIAL TREATMENTS

Lifestyle modifications for PMS/PMDD include dietary recommendations (ie, decreased caffeine, frequent snacks or meals, reduction of refined sugar and artificial sweeteners, and increase in complex carbohydrates) and exercise. Maintaining a steady serum glucose level with complex carbohydrates may decrease premenstrual food cravings and dysphoria and increase the availability of tryptophan in the brain for serotonin synthesis.[55] Exercise may improve premenstrual symptoms through an increase in beta-endorphin levels and improved well-being, but exercise has not yet been tested in women with prospectively confirmed PMS/PMDD.[86] Psychoeducation (ie, education about PMS, recommended diet and exercise regimens, self-monitoring, and other cognitive-behavioral techniques) has been reported superior to control conditions for reducing premenstrual symptoms.[87]

Reviews of cognitive-behavior therapy (CBT) have suggested weak but significant superiority to wait-list controls in reducing premenstrual symptoms, particularly mood and anxiety symptoms.[88–90] Efficacy of CBT may be due to modification of negative thoughts and increasing coping strategies. CBT may also have a role in decreasing emotional dysregulation.[91] A recent open study suggested that mindfulness-based stress reduction may be helpful for reducing symptoms of PMDD.[92]

SUMMARY

Women with severe PMS and PMDD comprise a substantial proportion of menstruating women. Once the diagnosis of severe PMS or PMDD is confirmed, an SSRI is considered first-line treatment and ovulation suppression second-line treatment.[12] SSRIs may be effective when administered daily or intermittently (from ovulation to menses or during symptomatic days).[56] Ovulation suppression options include ethinyl estradiol 20 μ/drospirenone 3 mg, possibly continuous use of OCs, transdermal estrogen, or GnRH agonists. Dietary changes, exercise, calcium, chasteberry, and cognitive therapy may be appropriate as first treatments in mild cases; otherwise, they may accompany medication treatment.[12] Future studies are needed to identify predictors for which women may benefit from SSRIs versus hormonal strategies, to examine the benefit of SSRIs combined with hormonal treatment, to determine the optimal duration for medication treatment, and to further investigate the role of psychosocial interventions.

REFERENCES

1. American Psychiatric Association. Diagnostic and statistical manual of mental disorders, Fifth Edition. Arlington (VA): American Psychiatric Association; 2013.
2. O'Brien PM, Backstrom T, Brown C, et al. Towards a consensus on diagnostic criteria, measurement and trial design of the premenstrual disorders: the ISPMD Montreal consensus. Arch Womens Ment Health 2011;14:13–21.
3. Epperson CN, Steiner M, Hartlage SA, et al. Premenstrual dysphoric disorder: evidence for a new category for DSM-5. Am J Psychiatry 2012;169:465–75.
4. Hartlage SA, Breaux CA, Yonkers KA. Addressing concerns about the inclusion of premenstrual dysphoric disorder in DSM-5. J Clin Psychiatry 2014;75:70–6.
5. Zachar P, Kendler KS. A diagnostic and statistical manual of mental disorders history of premenstrual dysphoric disorder. J Nerv Ment Dis 2014;202:346–52.
6. Browne TK. Is premenstrual dysphoric disorder really a disorder? J Bioeth Inq 2015;12:313–30.
7. Endicott J, Nee J, Harrison W. Daily record of severity of problems (DRSP): reliability and validity. Arch Womens Ment Health 2006;9:41–9.
8. Steiner M, Macdougall M, Brown E. The premenstrual symptoms screening tool (PSST) for clinicians. Arch Womens Ment Health 2003;6:203–9.
9. Steiner M, Peer M, Palova E, et al. The premenstrual symptoms screening tool revised for adolescents (PSST-A): prevalence of severe PMS and premenstrual dysphoric disorder in adolescents. Arch Womens Ment Health 2011;14:77–81.
10. Ismaili E, Walsh S, O'Brien PM, et al. Fourth consensus of the International Society for Premenstrual Disorders (ISPMD): auditable standards for diagnosis and management of premenstrual disorder. Arch Womens Ment Health 2016;19(6):953–8.
11. Rapkin AJ, Mikacich JA. Premenstrual dysphoric disorder and severe premenstrual syndrome in adolescents. Paediatr Drugs 2013;15:191–202.
12. Nevatte T, O'Brien PM, Backstrom T, et al. ISPMD consensus on the management of premenstrual disorders. Arch Womens Ment Health 2013;16:279–91.
13. Wittchen HU, Becker E, Lieb R, et al. Prevalence, incidence and stability of premenstrual dysphoric disorder in the community. Psychol Med 2002;32:119–32.

14. Merikangas KR, Foeldenyi M, Angst J. The Zurich Study. XIX. Patterns of menstrual disturbances in the community: results of the Zurich Cohort Study. Eur Arch Psychiatry Clin Neurosci 1993;243:23–32.
15. Halbreich U, Borenstein J, Pearlstein T, et al. The prevalence, impairment, impact, and burden of premenstrual dysphoric disorder (PMS/PMDD). Psychoneuroendocrinology 2003;28:1–23.
16. Heinemann LA, Minh TD, Heinemann K, et al. Intercountry assessment of the impact of severe premenstrual disorders on work and daily activities. Health Care Women Int 2012;33:109–24.
17. Kepple AL, Lee EE, Haq N, et al. History of postpartum depression in a clinic-based sample of women with premenstrual dysphoric disorder. J Clin Psychiatry 2016;77:e415–20.
18. Pilver CE, Levy BR, Libby DJ, et al. Posttraumatic stress disorder and trauma characteristics are correlates of premenstrual dysphoric disorder. Arch Womens Ment Health 2011;14:383–93.
19. Perkonigg A, Yonkers KA, Pfister H, et al. Risk factors for premenstrual dysphoric disorder in a community sample of young women: the role of traumatic events and posttraumatic stress disorder. J Clin Psychiatry 2004;65:1314–22.
20. Sassoon SA, Colrain IM, Baker FC. Personality disorders in women with severe premenstrual syndrome. Arch Womens Ment Health 2011;14:257–64.
21. Miller A, Vo H, Huo L, et al. Estrogen receptor alpha (ESR-1) associations with psychological traits in women with PMDD and controls. J Psychiatr Res 2010; 44:788–94.
22. Ducasse D, Jaussent I, Olie E, et al. Personality traits of suicidality are associated with premenstrual syndrome and premenstrual dysphoric disorder in a suicidal women sample. PLoS One 2016;11:e0148653.
23. Hong JP, Park S, Wang HR, et al. Prevalence, correlates, comorbidities, and suicidal tendencies of premenstrual dysphoric disorder in a nationwide sample of Korean women. Soc Psychiatry Psychiatr Epidemiol 2012;47:1937–45.
24. Pilver CE, Libby DJ, Hoff RA. Premenstrual dysphoric disorder as a correlate of suicidal ideation, plans, and attempts among a nationally representative sample. Soc Psychiatry Psychiatr Epidemiol 2013;48:437–46.
25. Buttner MM, Mott SL, Pearlstein T, et al. Examination of premenstrual symptoms as a risk factor for depression in postpartum women. Arch Womens Ment Health 2013;16:219–25.
26. Freeman EW, Sammel MD, Liu L, et al. Hormones and menopausal status as predictors of depression in women in transition to menopause. Arch Gen Psychiatry 2004;61:62–70.
27. Harlow BL, Cohen LS, Otto MW, et al. Prevalence and predictors of depressive symptoms in older premenopausal women: the Harvard Study of Moods and Cycles. Arch Gen Psychiatry 1999;56:418–24.
28. Richards M, Rubinow DR, Daly RC, et al. Premenstrual symptoms and perimenopausal depression. Am J Psychiatry 2006;163:133–7.
29. Schmidt PJ, Nieman LK, Danaceau MA, et al. Differential behavioral effects of gonadal steroids in women with and in those without premenstrual syndrome. N Engl J Med 1998;338:209–16.
30. Eser D, Schule C, Baghai TC, et al. Neuroactive steroids and affective disorders. Pharmacol Biochem Behav 2006;84:656–66.
31. Schule C, Nothdurfter C, Rupprecht R. The role of allopregnanolone in depression and anxiety. Prog Neurobiol 2014;113:79–87.

32. Mostallino MC, Mura ML, Maciocco E, et al. Changes in expression of the delta subunit of the GABA (A) receptor and in receptor function induced by progesterone exposure and withdrawal. J Neurochem 2006;99:321–32.
33. Timby E, Backstrom T, Nyberg S, et al. Women with premenstrual dysphoric disorder have altered sensitivity to allopregnanolone over the menstrual cycle compared to controls-a pilot study. Psychopharmacology (Berl) 2016;233: 2109–17.
34. Bengtsson SK, Nyberg S, Hedstrom H, et al. Isoallopregnanolone antagonize allopregnanolone-induced effects on saccadic eye velocity and self-reported sedation in humans. Psychoneuroendocrinology 2015;52:22–31.
35. Crowley SK, Girdler SS. Neurosteroid, GABAergic and hypothalamic pituitary adrenal (HPA) axis regulation: what is the current state of knowledge in humans? Psychopharmacology (Berl) 2014;231:3619–34.
36. Hantsoo L, Epperson CN. Premenstrual dysphoric disorder: epidemiology and treatment. Curr Psychiatry Rep 2015;17:87.
37. Martinez PE, Rubinow DR, Nieman LK, et al. 5α-reductase inhibition prevents the luteal phase increase in plasma allopregnanolone levels and mitigates symptoms in women with premenstrual dysphoric disorder. Neuropsychopharmacology 2016;41:1093–102.
38. Backstrom T, Bixo M, Johansson M, et al. Allopregnanolone and mood disorders. Prog Neurobiol 2014;113:88–94.
39. Schiller CE, Johnson SL, Abate AC, et al. Reproductive steroid regulation of mood and behavior. Compr Physiol 2016;6:1135–60.
40. Parry BL. The role of central serotonergic dysfunction in the aetiology of premenstrual dysphoric disorder: therapeutic implications. CNS Drugs 2001;15:277–85.
41. Yonkers KA, O'Brien PM, Eriksson E. Premenstrual syndrome. Lancet 2008;371: 1200–10.
42. Fanaei H, Khayat S, Kasaeian A, et al. Effect of curcumin on serum brain-derived neurotrophic factor levels in women with premenstrual syndrome: a randomized, double-blind, placebo-controlled trial. Neuropeptides 2016;56:25–31.
43. Marjoribanks J, Brown J, O'Brien PM, et al. Selective serotonin reuptake inhibitors for premenstrual syndrome. Cochrane Database Syst Rev 2013;(6):CD001396.
44. Guidotti A, Costa E. Can the antidysphoric and anxiolytic profiles of selective serotonin reuptake inhibitors be related to their ability to increase brain 3 alpha, 5 alpha-tetrahydroprogesterone (allopregnanolone) availability? Biol Psychiatry 1998;44:865–73.
45. Griffin LD, Mellon SH. Selective serotonin reuptake inhibitors directly alter activity of neurosteroidogenic enzymes. Proc Natl Acad Sci U S A 1999;96:13512–7.
46. Treloar SA, Heath AC, Martin NG. Genetic and environmental influences on premenstrual symptoms in an Australian twin sample. Psychol Med 2002;32:25–38.
47. Huo L, Straub RE, Schmidt PJ, et al. Risk for premenstrual dysphoric disorder is associated with genetic variation in ESR1, the estrogen receptor alpha gene. Biol Psychiatry 2007;62:925–33.
48. Magnay JL, El-Shourbagy M, Fryer AA, et al. Analysis of the serotonin transporter promoter rs25531 polymorphism in premenstrual dysphoric disorder. Am J Obstet Gynecol 2010;203:181.e1-e5.
49. Rubinow DR, Smith MJ, Schenkel LA, et al. Facial emotion discrimination across the menstrual cycle in women with premenstrual dysphoric disorder (PMDD) and controls. J Affect Disord 2007;104:37–44.
50. Protopopescu X, Tuescher O, Pan H, et al. Toward a functional neuroanatomy of premenstrual dysphoric disorder. J Affect Disord 2008;108:87–94.

51. Baller EB, Wei SM, Kohn PD, et al. Abnormalities of dorsolateral prefrontal function in women with premenstrual dysphoric disorder: a multimodal neuroimaging study. Am J Psychiatry 2013;170:305–14.
52. Comasco E, Sundstrom Poromaa I. Neuroimaging the menstrual cycle and premenstrual dysphoric disorder. Curr Psychiatry Rep 2015;17:77.
53. Halbreich U, O'Brien PMS, Eriksson E, et al. Are there differential symptom profiles that improve in response to different pharmacological treatments of premenstrual syndrome/premenstrual dysphoric disorder? CNS Drugs 2006;20:523–47.
54. Shah NR, Jones JB, Aperi J, et al. Selective serotonin reuptake inhibitors for premenstrual syndrome and premenstrual dysphoric disorder: a meta-analysis. Obstet Gynecol 2008;111:1175–82.
55. Pearlstein T. Psychotropic medications and other non-hormonal treatments for premenstrual disorders. Menopause Int 2012;18:60–4.
56. Steiner M, Li T. Luteal phase and symptom-onset dosing of SSRIs/SNRIs in the treatment of premenstrual dysphoria: clinical evidence and rationale. CNS Drugs 2013;27:583–9.
57. Steinberg EM, Cardoso GM, Martinez PE, et al. Rapid response to fluoxetine in women with premenstrual dysphoric disorder. Depress Anxiety 2012;29:531–40.
58. Yonkers KA, Kornstein SG, Gueorguieva R, et al. Symptom-onset dosing of sertraline for the treatment of premenstrual dysphoric disorder: a randomized clinical trial. JAMA Psychiatry 2015;72:1037–44.
59. Freeman EW, Sammel MD, Rickels K, et al. Clinical subtypes of premenstrual syndrome and responses to sertraline treatment. Obstet Gynecol 2011;118: 1293–300.
60. Freeman EW, Rickels K, Sammel MD, et al. Time to relapse after short- or long-term treatment of severe premenstrual syndrome with sertraline. Arch Gen Psychiatry 2009;66:537–44.
61. Joffe H, Petrillo LF, Viguera AC, et al. Treatment of premenstrual worsening of depression with adjunctive oral contraceptive pills: a preliminary report. J Clin Psychiatry 2007;68:1954–62.
62. Frey BN, Minuzzi L. Comorbid bipolar disorder and premenstrual dysphoric disorder: real patients, unanswered questions. Arch Womens Ment Health 2013;16: 79–81.
63. Lopez LM, Kaptein AA, Helmerhorst FM. Oral contraceptives containing drospirenone for premenstrual syndrome. Cochrane Database Syst Rev 2012;(2):CD006586.
64. Yonkers KA, Brown C, Pearlstein TB, et al. Efficacy of a new low-dose oral contraceptive with drospirenone in premenstrual dysphoric disorder. Obstet Gynecol 2005;106:492–501.
65. Pearlstein TB, Bachmann GA, Zacur HA, et al. Treatment of premenstrual dysphoric disorder with a new drospirenone-containing oral contraceptive formulation. Contraception 2005;72:414–21.
66. Freeman EW, Halbreich U, Grubb GS, et al. An overview of four studies of a continuous oral contraceptive (levonorgestrel 90 mcg/ethinyl estradiol 20 mcg) on premenstrual dysphoric disorder and premenstrual syndrome. Contraception 2012;85:437–45.
67. Halbreich U, Freeman EW, Rapkin AJ, et al. Continuous oral levonorgestrel/ethinyl estradiol for treating premenstrual dysphoric disorder. Contraception 2012;85: 19–27.
68. Wichianpitaya J, Taneepanichskul S. A comparative efficacy of low-dose combined oral contraceptives containing desogestrel and drospirenone in premenstrual symptoms. Obstet Gynecol Int 2013;2013:487143.

69. Wyatt KM, Dimmock PW, Ismail KM, et al. The effectiveness of GnRHa with and without 'add-back' therapy in treating premenstrual syndrome: a meta analysis. BJOG 2004;111:585–93.
70. Studd J. Treatment of premenstrual disorders by suppression of ovulation by transdermal estrogens. Menopause Int 2012;18:65–7.
71. Ford O, Lethaby A, Roberts H, et al. Progesterone for premenstrual syndrome. Cochrane Database Syst Rev 2012;(3):CD003415.
72. Nazari H, Yari F, Jariani M, et al. Premenstrual syndrome: a single-blind study of treatment with buspirone versus fluoxetine. Arch Gynecol Obstet 2013;287:469–72.
73. Sepede G, Martinotti G, Gambi F, et al. Lamotrigine augmentation in premenstrual dysphoric disorder: a case report. Clin Neuropharmacol 2013;36:31–3.
74. Kayatekin ZE, Sabo AN, Halbreich U. Levetiracetam for treatment of premenstrual dysphoric disorder: a pilot, open-label study. Arch Womens Ment Health 2008;11:207–11.
75. Jackson C, Pearson B, Girdler S, et al. Double-blind, placebo-controlled pilot study of adjunctive quetiapine SR in the treatment of PMS/PMDD. Hum Psychopharmacol 2015;30:425–34.
76. Thys-Jacobs S, Starkey P, Bernstein D, et al. Calcium carbonate and the premenstrual syndrome: effects on premenstrual and menstrual symptoms. Premenstrual Syndrome Study Group. Am J Obstet Gynecol 1998;179:444–52.
77. Yonkers KA, Pearlstein TB, Gotman N. A pilot study to compare fluoxetine, calcium and placebo in the treatment of premenstrual syndrome. J Clin Psychopharmacol 2013;33:614–20.
78. Shehata NA. Calcium versus oral contraceptive pills containing drospirenone for the treatment of mild to moderate premenstrual syndrome: a double blind randomized placebo controlled trial. Eur J Obstet Gynecol Reprod Biol 2016;198:100–4.
79. Wyatt KM, Dimmock PW, Jones PW, et al. Efficacy of vitamin B-6 in the treatment of premenstrual syndrome: systematic review. BMJ 1999;318:1375–81.
80. Whelan AM, Jurgens TM, Naylor H. Herbs, vitamins and minerals in the treatment of premenstrual syndrome: a systematic review. Can J Clin Pharmacol 2009;16:e407–29.
81. Dante G, Facchinetti F. Herbal treatments for alleviating premenstrual symptoms: a systematic review. J Psychosom Obstet Gynaecol 2011;32:42–51.
82. van Die MD, Burger HG, Teede HJ, et al. Vitex agnus-castus extracts for female reproductive disorders: a systematic review of clinical trials. Planta Med 2013;79:562–75.
83. Shechter A, Boivin DB. Sleep, hormones, and circadian rhythms throughout the menstrual cycle in healthy women and women with premenstrual dysphoric disorder. Int J Endocrinol 2010;2010:259345.
84. Parry BL, Meliska CJ, Sorenson DL, et al. Reduced phase-advance of plasma melatonin after bright morning light in the luteal, but not follicular, menstrual cycle phase in premenstrual dysphoric disorder: an extended study. Chronobiol Int 2011;28:415–24.
85. Kim SY, Park HJ, Lee H, et al. Acupuncture for premenstrual syndrome: a systematic review and meta-analysis of randomised controlled trials. BJOG 2011;118:899–915.
86. Daley A. Exercise and premenstrual symptomatology: a comprehensive review. J Womens Health 2009;18:895–9.

87. Taghizadeh Z, Shirmohammadi M, Feizi A, et al. The effect of cognitive behavioural psycho-education on premenstrual syndrome and related symptoms. J Psychiatr Ment Health Nurs 2013;20:705–13.
88. Busse JW, Montori VM, Krasnik C, et al. Psychological intervention for premenstrual syndrome: a meta-analysis of randomized controlled trials. Pyschother Psychosom 2009;78:6–15.
89. Lustyk MK, Gerrish WG, Shaver S, et al. Cognitive-behavioral therapy for premenstrual syndrome and premenstrual dysphoric disorder: a systematic review. Arch Womens Ment Health 2009;12:85–96.
90. Kleinstauber M, Witthoft M, Hiller W. Cognitive-behavioral and pharmacological interventions for premenstrual syndrome or premenstrual dysphoric disorder: a meta-analysis. J Clin Psychol Med Settings 2012;19:308–19.
91. Petersen N, London ED, Liang L, et al. Emotion regulation in women with premenstrual dysphoric disorder. Arch Womens Ment Health 2016;19(5):891–8.
92. Bluth K, Gaylord S, Nguyen K, et al. Mindfulness-based stress reduction as a promising intervention for amelioration of premenstrual dysphoric disorder symptoms. Mindfulness 2015;6:1292–302.

Psychopharmacology in Pregnancy and Breastfeeding

Jennifer L. Payne, MD

KEYWORDS

- Pregnancy • Breastfeeding • Antidepressants • Mood stabilizers
- Postpartum depression

KEY POINTS

- Many psychiatric medications can be taken safely during pregnancy and breastfeeding.
- There are significant risks associated with untreated psychiatric illness during pregnancy and postpartum.
- Many studies examining infant outcomes with exposure to psychotropic medications during pregnancy are confounded by illnesses, behaviors, and other risk factors associated with psychiatric illness.

WHY USE PSYCHIATRIC MEDICATIONS DURING PREGNANCY AND BREASTFEEDING?

Antepartum depression has been associated with low maternal weight gain,[1] increased rates of preterm birth,[1,2] low birth weight,[1] increased rates of cigarette, alcohol, and other substance use,[3] increased ambivalence about the pregnancy, and overall worse health status.[4] Children exposed to peripartum depression have higher cortisol levels than those of mothers not depressed,[5–8] and this continues through adolescence.[8] Importantly, maternal treatment of depression during pregnancy may help normalize infant cortisol levels.[9] Although the long-term effects of elevated cortisol are unclear, these findings may partially explain the mechanism for an increased vulnerability to psychopathology in children of antepartum depressed mothers.[10]

In turn, untreated antepartum depression is one of the strongest risk factors for postpartum depression (PPD),[11] and PPD has potentially devastating consequences, including suicide and infanticide. Suicides account for up to 20% of all postpartum deaths and represent one of the leading causes of peripartum mortality.[12] PPD has

This article originally appeared in the *Psychiatric Clinics of North America*, Volume 40, Issue 2, June 2017.
Dr J.L. Payne has performed legal consulting work for Pfizer, Astra Zeneca, Johnson and Johnson, and Eli Lilly. She has received research support from SAGE Therapeutics. She is currently receiving research support from the following NIH grants: R01 MH112704-01 and R01 MH 104262-01.
Johns Hopkins School of Medicine, 550 North Broadway, Suite 305, Baltimore, MD 21205, USA
E-mail address: Jpayne5@jhmi.edu

Med Clin N Am 103 (2019) 629–650
http://dx.doi.org/10.1016/j.mcna.2019.02.009
medical.theclinics.com

been associated with increased rates of infantile colic and impaired maternal-infant bonding.[13] PPD also interferes with parenting behavior, including less adequate infant safety and healthy child development practices,[14] such as the increased use of harsh discipline.[15] Finally, PPD has significant negative effects on infant development, including IQ, language, and behavior.[16]

Discontinuation of psychiatric medications for pregnancy is also associated with a high relapse rate of both major depression (MDD) and bipolar disorder (BD). Discontinuation of antidepressants in pregnant women with a history of MDD has been linked to relapse in 60% to 70% of women.[17,18] In women with BD, studies demonstrated a recurrence risk of 80% to 100% in pregnant women who discontinue mood stabilizers, whereas women who continued mood stabilizer treatment had a much lower risk of 29% to 37%.[19–21] Many women with psychiatric disorders experience relapse during pregnancy, both on and off medication. In one study, approximately 50% of women with a mood disorder reported significant mood symptoms during and/or after pregnancy.[22] Relapse then exposes the developing infant to the effects of untreated depression, which leads to adverse consequences for the woman, infant, and family.[1,23,24]

CONTROVERSIES AND LIMITATIONS OF THE LITERATURE

The treatment of psychiatric disorders during pregnancy is complicated by the fact that few studies have been conducted to determine which medications are efficacious, how changes in body weight and metabolism may affect dosing, and what alternatives to medications are available that successfully treat psychiatric illness during pregnancy. Thus, treatment decisions must be made with little hard data.

It is also important to understand that the use of psychotropic medications during pregnancy is essentially a "marker" for a population of women with different risk factors than the general population of pregnant women. These risk factors, including health-related behaviors, associated illnesses, and other characteristics, may influence the outcomes of studies attempting to examine the risks of in utero exposure of a psychotropic medication to a child. For example, diabetes, obesity, smoking, and substance use are more common in patients with psychiatric illness than in the general population. Studies that have not controlled for the underlying psychiatric illness and its confounding behaviors and characteristics may find associations between psychotropic medications and outcomes that are not directly caused by exposure to the medication itself, but by characteristics and behaviors that are more highly prevalent in the population of patients who take psychotropic medications during pregnancy.

US FOOD AND DRUG ADMINISTRATION PREGNANCY CATEGORIES AND THE PREGNANCY AND LACTATION LABELING RULE

In 2014, the US Food and Drug Administration (FDA) published the "Pregnancy and Lactation Labeling Rule," mandating changes to the content and format of prescription drug labeling detailing use during pregnancy and breastfeeding. The labeling changes went into effect in 2015 for all new products and will be phased in over time for older medications and products. The new labeling will attempt to summarize all currently available information to help the clinician weigh the risks and benefits of prescribing a drug during pregnancy or breastfeeding.

Because the new labeling will be phased in over time, it is still important to understand the meaning of the former FDA pregnancy categories. Categories include A, B, C, D, and X, and classification is based on the amount of evidence for safety in animal and human studies. Many clinicians assume that there is an increasing level of risk from category A to X, which is inaccurate. For example, medications that are category B simply have not been studied adequately in humans to warrant placing them into category A as safe or in C, D, or X, depending on the level of risk in humans. Most medications new to the market will therefore be placed in category B and should not necessarily be prescribed over older medications that are classified in category C or D, which at least have data regarding safety in pregnancy.

CLINICAL RECOMMENDATIONS FOR PSYCHIATRIC MEDICATION MANAGEMENT DURING PREGNANCY

Prepregnancy Planning

The ideal situation is to begin planning for pregnancy *before* pregnancy (**Box 1**). Ideally, the psychiatric treatment provider should assume that every woman of childbearing age will get pregnant and discuss whether the prescribed medications can be used safely during pregnancy and methods of birth control as part of her ongoing treatment. If a woman is taking a medication that should *not* be used during pregnancy unless absolutely necessary, such as valproic acid, a discussion should be held with the woman and, if possible, her partner to discuss this fact and to plan what should be done in case of accidental pregnancy. As many as 50% of pregnancies continue to be unplanned in the United States[25]; thus discussing ahead of time contingency plans for an unplanned pregnancy will minimize the chance that psychiatric medications will be abruptly discontinued and the patient will relapse.

Prepregnancy planning should be done ideally 6 to 12 months before attempting pregnancy so that there is enough time to make medication changes and ensure stability before pregnancy (see **Box 1**). Prepregnancy planning should take into account the patient's

1. Past psychiatric history,
2. Severity of illness,
3. Medication response history, and
4. Wishes and worries about treatment during pregnancy.

Box 1
Planning ahead: pregnancy in women with psychiatric disorders

- Encourage patient to have psychiatric care during and after pregnancy.
- All medication changes should be done before pregnancy if possible.
- Ideally the patient should be stable psychiatrically before attempting pregnancy.
- Use medications that something is known about: Older is usually (but not always) better.
- Minimize the number of exposures for the baby, including exposure to psychiatric illness.
- Consider breastfeeding when planning for pregnancy.
- If a baby was exposed to a medication during pregnancy, it may not make sense to discontinue the medication (or alternatively not breastfeed) for breastfeeding.
- Use a team approach—communicate with the family and other involved physicians frequently.
- Be supportive if the patient does not take your recommendations.
- FDA category B means *we do not have data in pregnancy in humans*—category B is not necessarily safer than category C or D.

Every case should be considered individually, and ultimately, there are no hard and fast rules—just the weighing of risks and benefits of the various options.

The patient and her partner's wishes regarding medication use during pregnancy should also be taken into account when designing the treatment plan. If one or the other is strongly against medication use during pregnancy, it is best for the treatment provider to make sure they understand the risks of no treatment and the rates of relapse and to outline a course of close follow-up during and after pregnancy, rather than insist on the use of medication during pregnancy. A partnership with good communication is important to maintain so that if there *is* a relapse of illness, the patient will remain safe and is more likely to seek care and treatment. Most important, the primary goal of treatment in pregnancy is to minimize the number of exposures. The goal is to not only minimize the number of medications but also limit exposure to psychiatric illness. If a woman is planning her pregnancy well in advance and she is on a newer, less-studied psychiatric medication, she and her provider can attempt to switch to a medication about which more safety data are available before pregnancy—but only if she does not have a history of nonresponse to that medication.

Unplanned Pregnancy

As noted, 50% of pregnancies are unplanned in the United States (**Box 2**).[25] Most practitioners will therefore have the experience at some point in their career of having a patient on psychiatric medications get pregnant unexpectedly. The principles outlined above for prepregnancy planning also apply in the case of an unplanned pregnancy. **Box 2** offers some additional tips on do's and don'ts in this situation. The most important principle to remember is: Do not stop all psychiatric medications precipitously in a knee-jerk reaction in response to the news of an unplanned pregnancy. This reaction can

a. Cause great stress and anxiety for the patient,
b. Precipitate discontinuation symptoms or withdrawal, and
c. Precipitate a relapse of mental illness.

The best approach is to review the medication list based on the principles outlined above for prepregnancy planning. Keep in mind that the baby is exposed already, and although stopping some medications may be necessary, doing so in a controlled and logical fashion is ideal. One common scenario is for a pregnant woman on a newer medication to receive the recommendation to switch to an older medication that

Box 2
Managing an unplanned pregnancy in women with psychiatric disorders

- See or talk to the patient as soon as possible.
- Do not stop all psychiatric medications immediately—most can be continued.
- If a decision is made to discontinue a medication, taper whenever possible.
- Consider stopping medications that are known to be teratogenic.
- As in prepregnancy planning, try to minimize the number of medications the patient is taking, but do so taking the patient's history into account, and remember that exposure to psychiatric illness counts as an exposure to the child.
- If the patient is psychiatrically ill, make a plan that includes treating the illness.

has more evidence for safety during pregnancy. Although this might have made sense before pregnancy, this plan would actually increase the exposures for the baby to the following:

1. The original medication;
2. The second medication;
3. Potential relapse.

If a decision is made to stop a medication, the medication should be tapered if at all possible. Tapering will eliminate the risk of withdrawal or discontinuation symptoms, thus maximizing outcomes for both the mother and the baby. It is also important to make a plan for treatment if the patient is psychiatrically ill. Many patients and practitioners overlook the fact that the patient may need more treatment, not less, in the excitement of an unplanned pregnancy.

Changes in Metabolism and Drug Clearance in Pregnancy

In pregnancy, major adaptive physiologic changes have a significant impact on the pharmacokinetic processes of drug absorption, distribution, metabolism, and excretion. Pregnancy's physiologic changes begin early and continue through the third trimester, resulting in an approximately 50% increase in plasma volume, increased body fat, and increased medication distribution volume. Renal blood flow, glomerular filtration rate, and medication elimination also increase,[26] and changes in liver enzyme activation occur (eg, CYP1A2 activity decreases; CYP2D6 and CYP3A activities increase).[27] These liver enzyme changes, which are mostly hormone dependent, can result in either increased or decreased medication clearance and are highly relevant to many psychotropic medications. Unfortunately, there are little data to help guide clinicians in decision making around medication dosing in pregnancy. When available, therapeutic monitoring of serum levels may help guide dosing. Otherwise, clinicians must rely on what is generally known regarding pharmacokinetic changes in pregnancy and some basic principles, including using the lowest beneficial dose of medication (ie, dose that provides sufficient maternal benefit while minimizing fetal exposure),[28] monitoring the woman's mental state frequently, and adjusting the medication dose as clinically indicated.[27]

General Recommendations for Breastfeeding

The benefits of breastfeeding for the baby are well documented, and the American Academy of Pediatrics advocates breastfeeding through the first 6 months of life. All psychotropic medications pass readily into breast milk. If an infant was exposed in utero to a psychiatric medication, it does not make sense to switch to another for breastfeeding. Exceptions include the following:

1. The mother's psychiatric illness has relapsed and the current medication regimen is not working;
2. The mother is on a medication that has a risk of severe side effects with continued exposure for the infant (for example, clozapine);
3. The infant appears to be having side effects or medical complications related to the medication exposure during breastfeeding.

If the medication regimen needs to be changed during breastfeeding, the patient and her treatment team should consider whether continued breastfeeding is worth the risks of increasing the number of exposures to medications for the infant.

It is important to involve the pediatrician in the decision-making process and to help monitor the baby for potential side effects. If the baby is being exposed to a medication that can be monitored via blood levels, then blood levels should be monitored in the baby intermittently and as needed. A common side effect for many psychiatric medications is sedation, and the baby should be monitored for excessive sleepiness and decreased feeding, particularly during the feeding after the mother takes the medication. If the baby is exposed to an antipsychotic medication, the baby should also be monitored for stiffness, cogwheeling, and extrapyramidal side effects, although these side effects are uncommon. At times it can be difficult to distinguish potential medication side effects from what is simply a fussy baby. When in doubt, the wisest choice is to do what makes the parents the most comfortable.

ANTIDEPRESSANTS

Antidepressants are the most commonly prescribed psychotropic medication during pregnancy.[29] The literature examining infant outcomes associated with antidepressant use during pregnancy is large and exemplifies the problem of "confounding by indication" found throughout this literature: several possible negative outcomes have been identified over the past 10 years by studies that did not control for the underlying psychiatric illness. However, subsequent more properly controlled studies have generally demonstrated either no or a very slight increased risk of adverse outcomes.

Overall, antidepressant use during pregnancy appears to be relatively safe. A small increase in the absolute risk of rare defects with selective serotonin reuptake inhibitor (SSRI) exposure was reported in one study,[30] but 4 meta-analyses examining the risk of major malformations with first-trimester SSRI exposure found no statistically significant increased risk.[31–34] Compared with the SSRIs, there are limited data for other types of antidepressants. Most studies examining the risk of tricyclic antidepressant exposure have found no increased risk of malformations,[35–39] although one large epidemiologic study found a significant increase in severe malformations (Odds Ratio: 1.36, 1.07–1.72).[40] Several studies of bupropion have found no association with major malformations.[41–43] The data available for other types of antidepressants are small but reassuring.[44,45]

The evolving literature examining in utero antidepressant exposure and infant cardiac defects is a good example of the importance of controlling for confounding factors in psychiatric clinical research. Some but not all previous studies demonstrated a possible association between in utero antidepressant (particularly SSRI) exposure and heart defects (reviewed in ref.[46]). However, most of these studies compared psychiatric population outcomes with the general population and did not control for risk factors and behaviors associated with MDD. More recent studies have done a better job of comparing "apples to apples" and have NOT found an association between antidepressant exposure and heart defects. For example, a recent study,[47] with a sample size of more than 900,000 women, did not find an association between first-trimester antidepressant exposure and cardiac malformations when the statistical analyses controlled for MDD by comparing the outcomes of women with MDD who took antidepressants to outcomes of women with MDD who did not take antidepressants. Another study[48] performed a meta-analysis of prospective cohort studies and found no association between SSRI use in the first trimester and heart defects when comparing women with MDD who took SSRIs in the first trimester with women with MDD who did not take antidepressants in pregnancy. Thus, the previously identified association between in utero antidepressant exposure and heart defects is likely associated with other risk factors and behaviors that are prevalent in the population of women with MDD.

A similar story has evolved for the possible association between in utero antidepressant exposure and persistent pulmonary hypertension in the newborn (PPHN). PPHN is a failure of the pulmonary vasculature to decrease resistance at birth, resulting in breathing difficulties for the infant, leading to hypoxia and often intubation, and carries a 10% to 20% mortality.[49] An association between SSRI exposure and PPHN was first noted in 2006[50] and led to an FDA alert and label change. Since this first study, 6 additional studies have been conducted: 3 found no association between SSRI exposure and PPHN[51–53] and 2 found an association,[54,55] although with lower odds ratios than the first study. The most recent[56] analyzed close to 3.8 million pregnancies and found no increased risk for PPHN when the analyses were adjusted for potential confounders associated with MDD.

In utero antidepressant exposure has been associated with low birth weight, premature birth, and most recently, autism. However, once again, studies that control for underlying confounds associated with psychiatric illness, in general, are negative. For example, a recent meta-analysis examined neonatal outcomes in women with MDD receiving no treatment and compared them with outcomes in women without MDD.[57] This study found that untreated depression was associated with significantly increased risks of preterm birth and low birth weight, indicating that exposure to the illness MDD affected infant outcomes. A similar story is currently developing for the literature examining in utero antidepressant exposure and autism. A recent systematic review and meta-analysis found that maternal psychiatric illness is a "major confounding factor" in the association between SSRI exposure and autism and that there was no an increased risk for autism when analyses controlled for maternal psychiatric illness.[58]

Although the studies in this area are also plagued with lack of controlling for the underlying psychiatric illness and associated risk factors, the overall results suggest that the use of antidepressants in early pregnancy may be associated with a modestly increased risk of spontaneous abortion with odds ratios in the range of 1.4 to 1.6.[45,59–62]

One other outcome that does appear to be associated with in utero antidepressant exposure is poor neonatal adaptation syndrome (PNAS), a transient cluster of symptoms seen in newborns. The first report of "withdrawal" symptoms in babies exposed to antidepressants occurred in 1973.[63] It is unclear if PNAS is actually a result of "withdrawal" from the antidepressant or is due to toxicity or even a combination of both. There are several limitations in the available literature, including inconsistent definitions, no standardized measurement tool, a lack of blinded ratings, and a lack of studies investigating treatment or prevention of the syndrome as well as long-term outcomes. The FDA instituted a class labeling change in 2004 for both SSRI and SNRI (serotonin-norepinephrine reuptake inhibitors) antidepressants warning that third-trimester exposure may be associated with PNAS. According to the label change, "reported clinical findings have included respiratory distress, cyanosis, apnea, seizures, temperature instability, feeding difficulty, vomiting, hypoglycemia, hypotonia, hypertonia, hyperreflexia, tremor, jitteriness, irritability, and constant crying" and recommend considering tapering of the antidepressant before delivery. This recommendation has not, to date, been subjected to evidence-based testing, and it currently remains unclear if this practice decreases the risk for PNAS or is safe for the mother. Most cases of the PNAS appear to be mild and self-limited and have not been associated with lasting repercussions.[64] Available data suggest that approximately one-third of exposed infants will have at least mild symptoms consistent with the syndrome and this risk increases when multiple agents, particularly benzodiazepines, are used.[65] Clearly, larger, more rigorous studies of the syndrome as well as strategies to minimize the risk of PNAS are needed. At this time, there is simply not enough evidence from a safety perspective to recommend tapering of antidepressants in the third trimester, particularly in cases of moderate to severe maternal mental illness. In fact, many women may need higher doses in the third trimester, because pharmacokinetic changes and an increased volume of distribution can lead to lower drug concentrations and a re-emergence of symptoms.

In general, antidepressant use during breastfeeding is considered safe with most studies demonstrating low or undetectable blood levels.[66] Infants should be monitored for sedation, difficulty feeding, and difficulty sleeping, although these side effects are uncommon.

MOOD STABILIZERS

In general, valproic acid and carbamazepine should not be used during pregnancy because of high rates of malformation associated with these medications. Valproic acid is associated with as much as a 10% rate of malformations with first-trimester exposure, including neural tube defects, effects on cognition and brain volume, craniofacial anomalies, cardiac defects, cleft palate, and hypospadias[62] and may be linked to autism.[67,68] Carbamazepine also carries an increased risk of malformations, primarily of spina bifida as well as other neural tube defects, facial abnormalities, skeletal abnormalities, hypospadias, and diaphragmatic hernia.[62] Carbamazepine is also a competitive inhibitor of prothrombin precursors and may increase the risk of neonatal hemorrhage. Providers should encourage pregnant women who elect to continue any anticonvulsant to take high-dose folate (4 mg per day) for the theoretic benefit of reducing the risk of neural tube defects and to undergo a second-trimester ultrasound to screen for major congenital anomalies. In contrast to pregnancy, both valproic acid and carbamazepine are considered safe during breastfeeding.[66]

There appears to be no increased risk of congenital defects above the baseline risk with lamotrigine monotherapy.[69] An early study found a possible increased risk of cleft palate defects.[70] However, a more recent and larger study using a population-based case-control design using data from the EUROCAT congenital malformation registries, which included data on 3.9 million births, did not find an increased risk of cleft palate.[71] Lamotrigine levels may decrease over the course of pregnancy and thus should be followed and adjusted if needed.[72] Lamotrigine is also considered safe in breastfeeding.[66]

Lithium use during the first trimester has been associated with an increased risk of a serious congenital heart defect known as Ebstein anomaly. The risk for Ebstein anomaly with first-trimester exposure was originally thought to be much higher (400 times higher than baseline), but a pooled analysis of lithium-exposed pregnancies found that this defect only occurs in less than 1% of exposed children.[73] Lithium has also been associated with perinatal toxicity, including case reports of hypotonia, cyanosis, neonatal goiter, and diabetes insipidus. For women with severe BD, the risk of recurrence during pregnancy may overshadow the relatively small risk of Ebstein anomaly. On the other hand, for women with significant periods of euthymia and few past mood episodes, slowly tapering off lithium and reintroducing lithium after the first trimester may help reduce the risk of relapse. There are limited data on the long-term outcomes of children exposed in utero, but a follow-up of children up to age 5 demonstrated no evidence of cognitive or behavioral issues in a small sample of children.[74] Lithium levels should be followed closely during pregnancy, and the dose should be held with the initiation of labor. Hydration during delivery should be maintained and the dosage reduced to prepregnancy levels (if increased during pregnancy) with close monitoring of serum levels.[62] Breastfeeding while taking lithium can be tricky due to the risk of elevated lithium levels in a dehydrated baby. A recent report demonstrated relatively low levels of lithium in breastfeeding infants, but the sample size was small.[75] If a woman breastfeeds while taking lithium, levels should be monitored periodically in the baby, and there should be a low threshold for taking the infant to the emergency room (ER) in the setting of dehydration (such as a gastrointestinal illness).

ANTIPSYCHOTICS

Overall, it appears that antipsychotics are, for the most part, relatively safe to use in pregnancy and that *not* using these medications when indicated for serious mental illness poses a much greater risk, including suicide and infanticide.[76] For example, a study that examined birth outcomes in a matched cohort of women who used antipsychotics in pregnancy (n = 1021) and who did not (n = 1021), and an unmatched cohort of women who used antipsychotics in pregnancy (n = 1200) and who did not (n = 40,000), revealed an increased risk of adverse outcomes in the unmatched cohort only indicating that the psychiatric illness itself, not the use of antipsychotics, increased the risk of adverse outcomes for the infant.[77] Quetiapine, risperidone, haloperidol, and olanzapine exhibit the lowest placental transfer from mother to fetus.[78]

Normal metabolic changes in pregnancy may increase the risk for gestational diabetes in conjunction with the use of antipsychotics. In fact, many antipsychotics are associated with excessive maternal weight gain, increased infant birth weight, and increased risk of gestational diabetes.[78–80] Routine ultrasound monitoring of fetal size in late pregnancy for women taking these medications is warranted.[80,81] Several studies suggest increased risk of hyperglycemia associated with the use of atypical antipsychotics in pregnancy.[82] However, this may be due to higher baseline rates of diabetes in women prescribed antipsychotics,[77,83] reinforcing the need for a thorough evaluation and appropriate glucose monitoring for women prescribed these medications.

There is a lack of evidence regarding late pregnancy exposure to antipsychotics, including little on longer-term developmental outcomes, and so the risks remain unclear. Behaviors observed in infants exposed to antipsychotics in utero include motor restlessness, dystonia, hypertonia, and tremor.[84,85] In 2011, the FDA issued a drug safety communication for all antipsychotics regarding the potential risks of abnormal muscle movements and withdrawal symptoms in exposed infants.[86] The few studies examining the relationship between in utero exposure to older "typical" antipsychotics and neurodevelopment have shown no difference in IQ or behavioral functioning at 5 years.[87–89] In contrast, studies of the newer atypical antipsychotics have shown associated neurodevelopmental delays at 6 months of age[90,91] that are no longer evident at 12 months.[62,90]

Antipsychotic levels in breast milk have generally been found to be low, but there is a significant lack of data on long-term outcomes and potential side effects, including effects on development and extrapyramidal side effects.[66] Women should be counseled regarding this lack of data, and exposed infants should be monitored carefully by their pediatrician.

ANTIANXIETY AGENTS

Studies of benzodiazepine use during pregnancy have been contradictory. Benzodiazepine use during pregnancy has been associated with case reports of perinatal toxicity, including temperature dysregulation, apnea, depressed APGAR scores, hypotonia, and poor feeding. In addition, early studies revealed an elevated risk of oral cleft palate defects. However, more recent studies have shown that the overall risk of cleft lip and palate with benzodiazepine use in pregnancy is likely quite low.[92,93] Infants exposed to an SSRI in combination with a benzodiazepine may have a higher incidence of congenital heart defects even when controlling for maternal illness characteristics.[94] Shorter-acting agents are preferred for breastfeeding to limit sedating side effects in the infant.[66]

In general, although not approved for the treatment of anxiety, gabapentin is considered a safe alternative for the management of anxiety symptoms during pregnancy. Several studies have indicated that there is no increased risk of major congenital malformations with gabapentin,[95,96] although a recent study found a higher rate of preterm birth, low birth weight, and need for neonatal intensive care admission.[97] Like gabapentin, pregabalin is not approved for the treatment of anxiety but clinically has some utility in decreasing anxiety symptoms. It is less studied than gabapentin, but there is no known association with an increased risk of malformations.

Buspirone is also useful for anxiety; animal studies have not demonstrated evidence of teratogenesis, but there is no available evidence in humans.

In considering the risks and benefits of antianxiety agents use during pregnancy, clinicians should also consider the risks of untreated insomnia and anxiety in pregnancy, which may lead to physiologic effects as well as diminished self-care, worsening mood, and impaired functioning. Given the consequences of untreated psychiatric symptoms to both women and children and the limited risks associated with antianxiety agent use, some women with overwhelming anxiety symptoms or sleep disturbance may find that the benefits outweigh any theoretic risks.

STIMULANTS

The data regarding stimulant exposure in pregnancy and lactation are sparse and plagued by small numbers and polypharmacy. For many women, the lack of knowledge about safety in pregnancy and lactation supports discontinuation of stimulants, which are typically prescribed for attention-deficit/hyperactivity disorder or as an adjunctive medication. To date, there is no evidence of increased organ malformations,[98] although there may be an increased risk of spontaneous abortion.[99,100]

SUMMARY

Although growing, the data regarding the safety of psychiatric medications during pregnancy and lactation (**Table 1**) continue to be limited, primarily by studies that have not properly controlled for the risk factors and behaviors that are more common in the psychiatric population that may influence pregnancy outcomes. Most well-controlled studies are reassuring to date, especially for antidepressants. Areas that need further research include the safety of antipsychotics in pregnancy and breastfeeding and long-term outcomes for children exposed to psychiatric medications. The area will also benefit from studies that examine the issue of dosing of psychiatric medications in pregnancy and prevention of recurrent illness both in and after pregnancy. One fact that is clear from the available literature is that psychiatric illness is associated with negative outcomes for both mother and child and should be actively clinically managed despite the lack of data.

Table 1
Psychiatric medications in pregnancy and breastfeeding

Medication	FDA Category	Potential Complications	Pregnancy Recommendations	Breastfeeding Recommendations
Antidepressants				
SSRIs	Citalopram = C Escitalopram = C Fluoxetine = C Fluvoxamine = C Paroxetine = D Sertraline = C Vilazodone = C	• Modest increased risk of spontaneous abortion • Modest increased risk of preterm birth and low birth weight but may be secondary to psychiatric illness • No confirmed risk of birth defects except for small absolute increased risk of cardiac defects (2/1000 births) with *paroxetine* with first-trimester exposure • PNAS with third-trimester exposure in about 30% of cases • Conflicting evidence for small increased risk of persistent pulmonary hypertension with third-trimester exposure (may be secondary to psychiatric illness)	• Best studied class of antidepressants • Most studies confounded by indication (ie, not controlled for the underlying psychiatric illness) • Behaviors and risk factors associated with the psychiatric illness might influence some of the associations • Large studies that attempt to control for the underlying psychiatric illness generally suggest no increased risks • High relapse rate in women who stop their antidepressants for pregnancy • Avoid use of paroxetine during pregnancy if possible	• Generally considered safe

(*continued on next page*)

Table 1
(*continued*)

Medication	FDA Category	Potential Complications	Pregnancy Recommendations	Breastfeeding Recommendations
Serotonin and norepinephrine reuptake inhibitors	Duloxetine = C Desvenlafaxine = C Venlafaxine = C	• Less data available • Modest increased risk of spontaneous abortion • Modest increased risk of preterm birth and low birth weight but may be secondary to psychiatric illness • No confirmed risk of birth defects • PNAS with third-trimester exposure • Conflicting evidence for small absolute increased risk of persistent pulmonary hypertension with third-trimester exposure (may be secondary to psychiatric illness)	• Most studies are confounded by not controlling for the underlying psychiatric illness	• Generally considered safe
Other antidepressants	Buproprion = C Mirtazapine = C Trazodone = C	• Less data available • Modestly increased risk of spontaneous abortion • Modest increased risk of preterm birth and low birth weight but may be secondary to psychiatric illness • No confirmed risk of birth defects • PNAS with third-trimester exposure • Conflicting evidence for small absolute increased risk of persistent pulmonary hypertension with third-trimester exposure (may be secondary to psychiatric illness)	• Most studies are confounded by not controlling for the underlying psychiatric illness	• Generally considered safe

Tricyclic antidepressants	Amitriptyline = C Clomipramine = C Desipramine = N Doxepin = N Imipramine = N Nortriptyline = N	• Less data available • Modestly increased risk of spontaneous abortion • Modest increased risk of preterm birth and low birth weight but may be secondary to psychiatric illness • No confirmed risk of birth defects • PNAS with third-trimester exposure • Conflicting evidence for small absolute increased risk of persistent pulmonary hypertension with third-trimester exposure (may be secondary to psychiatric illness)	• Therapeutic drug monitoring allows monitoring of serum levels and appropriate dose adjustments during pregnancy	• Generally considered safe except for doxepin • Monitor the baby for sedation • May get levels in the infant
Monoamine oxidase inhibitors	Selegiline transdermal = C Phenelzine = C Tranylcypromine = N	• Much less data available • Modest increased risk of spontaneous abortion • Modest increased risk of preterm birth and low birth weight but may be secondary to psychiatric illness • No confirmed risk of birth defects • PNAS with third-trimester exposure (little data) • Unstudied with persistent pulmonary hypertension	• Orthostatic hypotension may be pronounced in pregnancy	• Little to no data
Mood Stabilizers				
Lamotrigine	C	• No increased risk of major congenital malformations • One early and small study found an association with cleft palate that has not been replicated	• Serum levels should be monitored and maintained during pregnancy as levels usually decrease as pregnancy progresses	• Considered safe

(continued on next page)

Table 1
(continued)

Medication	FDA Category	Potential Complications	Pregnancy Recommendations	Breastfeeding Recommendations
Valproic acid	D	• Associated with up to 10% rate of malformations. Neural tube defects, effects on cognition and brain volume, craniofacial anomalies, cardiac defects, cleft palate, and hypospadias have been described • Recently linked to autism	• Generally should not be used during pregnancy • High-dose folate (4 mg) supplementation is recommended	• Considered safe
Carbamazepine	D	• Increased risk of malformations, including spina bifida, other neural tube defects, facial abnormalities, skeletal abnormalities, hypospadias, and diaphragmatic hernia • Increased the risk of neonatal hemorrhage	• Generally should not be used during pregnancy • High-dose folate (4 mg) supplementation is recommended	• Considered safe
Lithium	D	• 1/1000 develop Ebstein anomaly • No cognitive or behavioral effects in exposed children	• Lithium levels should be followed closely during pregnancy • The dose should be held or reduced with the initiation of labor • Postpartum, the dose should be reduced to prepregnancy levels (if it was increased during pregnancy) • Fetal echocardiogram in the first trimester is recommended	• Should only be used in breastfeeding with close monitoring of infant blood levels • If infant becomes dehydrated, must go to the ER for hydration and lithium level

Antipsychotic Medications				
Typical antipsychotics	Chlorpromazine = N Fluphenazine = N Haloperidol = C Loxapine = N Perphenazine = C Trifluoperazine = C Thiothixene = N Fluphenazine = N	• No major congenital malformations have been demonstrated • Associated with low birth weight and preterm delivery • No difference in IQ or behavior in exposed children • Exposure in third trimester associated with transient extrapyramidal and withdrawal symptoms in the infant	• Most studies are confounded by not controlling for the underlying psychiatric illness • High-potency antipsychotics are preferred over low potency due to anticholinergic, hypotensive, and antihistaminergic side effects	• Limited to no data on long-term outcomes for exposed infants • Considered relatively safe • More studies on short-term and long-term side effects and developmental outcomes need to be done; monitor for extrapyramidal side effects and sedation
Atypical antipsychotics	Aripiprazole = C Asenapine = C Clozapine = B Lurasadone = B Olanzapine = C Paliperidone = C Quetiapine = C Risperidone = C Ziprasidone = C	• No major congenital malformations have been demonstrated • May increase maternal weight gain • May increase risk of gestational diabetes • May increase size of the baby • Neurodevelopmental delays found at 6 mo but resolved by 12 mo	• Most studies are confounded by indication (ie, not controlled for the underlying psychiatric illness) • There are less data available for clozapine and Lurasadone • Glucose monitoring recommended • Routine ultrasound monitoring of fetal size in late pregnancy should be obtained • Clozapine has been associated with floppy baby syndrome and exposed infants should be monitored for agranulocytosis weekly for 6 mo	• Limited to no data on long-term outcomes for exposed infants • Considered relatively safe • More studies on short-term and long-term side effects and developmental outcomes need to be done • Monitor for extrapyramidal side effects and sedation • Do not use clozapine in breastfeeding

(*continued on next page*)

Table 1
(continued)

Medication	FDA Category	Potential Complications	Pregnancy Recommendations	Breastfeeding Recommendations
Antianxiety Medications				
Benzodiazepines	Alprazolam = D Chlordiazepoxide = D Clonazepam = D Diazepam = D Lorazepam = D Oxazepam = D	• May induce perinatal toxicity: temperature dysregulation, apnea, lower APGAR scores, hypotonia, and poor feeding • Use just before delivery associated with floppy baby syndrome • Some studies suggest oral cleft palate defects; others are negative	• Consider tapering benzodiazepines before delivery • Intermittent use is unlikely to induce withdrawal symptoms in the newborn	• Use during breastfeeding may cause sedation or potential infant dependence • Shorter-acting agents preferred
Gabapentin	C	• No increased risk of major congenital malformations • One study found increased risk of preterm birth, low birth weight, and neonatal intensive care unit admission	• Generally considered safe in pregnancy	• Considered moderately safe • Monitor for sedation
Pregabalin	C	• Evidence of congenital malformations and growth restriction in animals • No evidence of congenital malformations in humans, but there are few studies	• Generally considered safe in pregnancy • Less data than gabapentin	• Limited data on passage into breast milk • Monitor for sedation • Another medication may be preferred
Buspirone	B	• No evidence of congenital malformations in animals • No data in humans	• No data	• No data • No reports of adverse events
Adjunctive Medications				
Stimulants	Amphetamine = C Dextroamphetamine = C Lisdexamfetamine = C Methylphenidate = C	• Decreased fetal survival in rats • Possible increased risk of spontaneous abortion and miscarriage • No evidence of major congenital malformations	• Most studies are complicated by polypharmacy and/or substance abuse as well as confounding by indication • Most studies have small samples	• No long-term studies • No reports of adverse events

REFERENCES

1. Yonkers KA, Wisner KL, Stewart DE, et al. The management of depression during pregnancy: a report from the American Psychiatric Association and the American College of Obstetricians and Gynecologists. Gen Hosp Psychiatry 2009;31(5):403–13.
2. Li D, Liu L, Odouli R. Presence of depressive symptoms during early pregnancy and the risk of preterm delivery: a prospective cohort study. Hum Reprod 2009; 24(1):146–53.
3. Zuckerman B, Amaro H, Bauchner H, et al. Depressive symptoms during pregnancy: relationship to poor health behaviors. Am J Obstet Gynecol 1989;160(5 Pt 1):1107–11.
4. Orr ST, Blazer DG, James SA, et al. Depressive symptoms and indicators of maternal health status during pregnancy. J Womens Health (Larchmt) 2007; 16(4):535–42.
5. Ashman SB, Dawson G, Panagiotides H, et al. Stress hormone levels of children of depressed mothers. Dev Psychopathol 2002;14(2):333–49.
6. Diego MA, Field T, Hernandez-Reif M, et al. Prepartum, postpartum, and chronic depression effects on newborns. Psychiatry 2004;67(1):63–80.
7. Essex MJ, Klein MH, Cho E, et al. Maternal stress beginning in infancy may sensitize children to later stress exposure: effects on cortisol and behavior. Biol Psychiatry 2002;52(8):776–84.
8. Halligan SL, Herbert J, Goodyer IM, et al. Exposure to postnatal depression predicts elevated cortisol in adolescent offspring. Biol Psychiatry 2004;55(4): 376–81.
9. Brennan PA, Pargas R, Walker EF, et al. Maternal depression and infant cortisol: influences of timing, comorbidity and treatment. J Child Psychol Psychiatry 2008;49(10):1099–107.
10. O'Connor TG, Ben-Shlomo Y, Heron J, et al. Prenatal anxiety predicts individual differences in cortisol in pre-adolescent children. Biol Psychiatry 2005;58(3): 211–7.
11. Robertson E, Grace S, Wallington T, et al. Antenatal risk factors for postpartum depression: a synthesis of recent literature. Gen Hosp Psychiatry 2004;26(4): 289–95.
12. Lindahl V, Pearson JL, Colpe L. Prevalence of suicidality during pregnancy and the postpartum. Arch Womens Ment Health 2005;8(2):77–87.
13. Akman I, Kuscu K, Ozdemir N, et al. Mothers' postpartum psychological adjustment and infantile colic. Arch Dis Child 2006;91(5):417–9.
14. Flynn HA, Davis M, Marcus SM, et al. Rates of maternal depression in pediatric emergency department and relationship to child service utilization. Gen Hosp Psychiatry 2004;26(4):316–22.
15. McLearn KT, Minkovitz CS, Strobino DM, et al. The timing of maternal depressive symptoms and mothers' parenting practices with young children: implications for pediatric practice. Pediatrics 2006;118(1):e174–82.
16. Grace SL, Evindar A, Stewart DE. The effect of postpartum depression on child cognitive development and behavior: a review and critical analysis of the literature. Arch Womens Ment Health 2003;6(4):263–74.
17. Cohen LS, Altshuler LL, Harlow BL, et al. Relapse of major depression during pregnancy in women who maintain or discontinue antidepressant treatment. JAMA 2006;295(5):499–507.

18. Cohen LS, Nonacs RM, Bailey JW, et al. Relapse of depression during pregnancy following antidepressant discontinuation: a preliminary prospective study. Arch Womens Ment Health 2004;7(4):217–21.
19. Viguera AC, Nonacs R, Cohen LS, et al. Risk of recurrence of bipolar disorder in pregnant and nonpregnant women after discontinuing lithium maintenance. Am J Psychiatry 2000;157(2):179–84.
20. Viguera AC, Whitfield T, Baldessarini RJ, et al. Risk of recurrence in women with bipolar disorder during pregnancy: prospective study of mood stabilizer discontinuation. Am J Psychiatry 2007;164(12):1817–24 [quiz: 1923].
21. Newport DJ, Stowe ZN, Viguera AC, et al. Lamotrigine in bipolar disorder: efficacy during pregnancy. Bipolar Disord 2008;10(3):432–6.
22. Payne JL, Roy PS, Murphy-Eberenz K, et al. Reproductive cycle-associated mood symptoms in women with major depression and bipolar disorder. J Affect Disord 2007;99(1–3):221–9.
23. Murray L, Sinclair D, Cooper P, et al. The socioemotional development of 5-year-old children of postnatally depressed mothers. J Child Psychol Psychiatry 1999; 40(8):1259–71.
24. Marmorstein NR, Malone SM, Iacono WG. Psychiatric disorders among offspring of depressed mothers: associations with paternal psychopathology. Am J Psychiatry 2004;161(9):1588–94.
25. Mosher WD, Bachrach CA. Understanding U.S. fertility: continuity and change in the National Survey of Family Growth, 1988-1995. Fam Plann Perspect 1996;28(1):4–12.
26. Seeman MV. Gender differences in the prescribing of antipsychotic drugs. Am J Psychiatry 2004;161(8):1324–33.
27. Tracy TS, Venkataramanan R, Glover DD, et al. Temporal changes in drug metabolism (CYP1A2, CYP2D6 and CYP3A activity) during pregnancy. Am J Obstet Gynecol 2005;192(2):633–9.
28. DeVane CL, Stowe ZN, Donovan JL, et al. Therapeutic drug monitoring of psychoactive drugs during pregnancy in the genomic era: challenges and opportunities. J Psychopharmacol 2006;20(4 Suppl):54–9.
29. Hanley GE, Oberlander TF. The effect of perinatal exposures on the infant: antidepressants and depression. Best Pract Res Clin Obstet Gynaecol 2014;28(1): 37–48.
30. Alwan S, Reefhuis J, Rasmussen SA, et al. Patterns of antidepressant medication use among pregnant women in a United States population. J Clin Pharmacol 2011;51(2):264–70.
31. Rahimi R, Nikfar S, Abdollahi M. Pregnancy outcomes following exposure to serotonin reuptake inhibitors: a meta-analysis of clinical trials. Reprod Toxicol 2006;22(4):571–5.
32. Addis A, Koren G. Safety of fluoxetine during the first trimester of pregnancy: a meta-analytical review of epidemiological studies. Psychol Med 2000;30(1): 89–94.
33. Einarson TR, Einarson A. Newer antidepressants in pregnancy and rates of major malformations: a meta-analysis of prospective comparative studies. Pharmacoepidemiol Drug Saf 2005;14(12):823–7.
34. O'Brien L, Einarson TR, Sarkar M, et al. Does paroxetine cause cardiac malformations? J Obstet Gynaecol Can 2008;30(8):696–701.
35. Davis RL, Rubanowice D, McPhillips H, et al. Risks of congenital malformations and perinatal events among infants exposed to antidepressant medications during pregnancy. Pharmacoepidemiol Drug Saf 2007;16(10):1086–94.

36. Nulman I, Rovet J, Stewart DE, et al. Neurodevelopment of children exposed in utero to antidepressant drugs. N Engl J Med 1997;336(4):258–62.
37. Pastuszak A, Schick-Boschetto B, Zuber C, et al. Pregnancy outcome following first-trimester exposure to fluoxetine (Prozac). JAMA 1993;269(17):2246–8.
38. Simon GE, Cunningham ML, Davis RL. Outcomes of prenatal antidepressant exposure. Am J Psychiatry 2002;159(12):2055–61.
39. Ramos E, St-Andre M, Rey E, et al. Duration of antidepressant use during pregnancy and risk of major congenital malformations. Br J Psychiatry 2008;192(5): 344–50.
40. Reis M, Kallen B. Delivery outcome after maternal use of antidepressant drugs in pregnancy: an update using Swedish data. Psychol Med 2010;40(10): 1723–33.
41. Chun-Fai-Chan B, Koren G, Fayez I, et al. Pregnancy outcome of women exposed to bupropion during pregnancy: a prospective comparative study. Am J Obstet Gynecol 2005;192(3):932–6.
42. Cole JA, Modell JG, Haight BR, et al. Bupropion in pregnancy and the prevalence of congenital malformations. Pharmacoepidemiol Drug Saf 2007;16(5): 474–84.
43. Alwan S, Reefhuis J, Botto LD, et al. Maternal use of bupropion and risk for congenital heart defects. Am J Obstet Gynecol 2010;203(1):52.e1-6.
44. Byatt N, Deligiannidis KM, Freeman MP. Antidepressant use in pregnancy: a critical review focused on risks and controversies. Acta Psychiatr Scand 2013;127(2):94–114.
45. Yonkers KA, Blackwell KA, Glover J, et al. Antidepressant use in pregnant and postpartum women. Annu Rev Clin Psychol 2014;10:369–92.
46. Chisolm MS, Payne JL. Management of psychotropic drugs during pregnancy. BMJ 2016;532:h5918.
47. Huybrechts KF, Palmsten K, Avorn J, et al. Antidepressant use in pregnancy and the risk of cardiac defects. N Engl J Med 2014;370(25):2397–407.
48. Wang S, Yang L, Wang L, et al. Selective serotonin reuptake inhibitors (SSRIs) and the risk of congenital heart defects: a meta-analysis of prospective cohort studies. J Am Heart Assoc 2015;4(5).
49. Walsh-Sukys MC, Tyson JE, Wright LL, et al. Persistent pulmonary hypertension of the newborn in the era before nitric oxide: practice variation and outcomes. Pediatrics 2000;105(1 Pt 1):14–20.
50. Chambers CD, Hernandez-Diaz S, Van Marter LJ, et al. Selective serotonin-reuptake inhibitors and risk of persistent pulmonary hypertension of the newborn. N Engl J Med 2006;354(6):579–87.
51. Andrade SE, McPhillips H, Loren D, et al. Antidepressant medication use and risk of persistent pulmonary hypertension of the newborn. Pharmacoepidemiol Drug Saf 2009;18(3):246–52.
52. Wichman CL, Moore KM, Lang TR, et al. Congenital heart disease associated with selective serotonin reuptake inhibitor use during pregnancy. Mayo Clin Proc 2009;84(1):23–7.
53. Wilson KL, Zelig CM, Harvey JP, et al. Persistent pulmonary hypertension of the newborn is associated with mode of delivery and not with maternal use of selective serotonin reuptake inhibitors. Am J Perinatol 2011;28(1):19–24.
54. Kallen B, Olausson PO. Maternal use of selective serotonin re-uptake inhibitors and persistent pulmonary hypertension of the newborn. Pharmacoepidemiol Drug Saf 2008;17(8):801–6.

55. Kieler H, Artama M, Engeland A, et al. Selective serotonin reuptake inhibitors during pregnancy and risk of persistent pulmonary hypertension in the newborn: population based cohort study from the five Nordic countries. BMJ 2012;344: d8012.
56. Huybrechts KF, Bateman BT, Palmsten K, et al. Antidepressant use late in pregnancy and risk of persistent pulmonary hypertension of the newborn. JAMA 2015;313(21):2142–51.
57. Jarde A, Morais M, Kingston D, et al. Neonatal outcomes in women with untreated antenatal depression compared with women without depression: a systematic review and meta-analysis. JAMA Psychiatry 2016;73(8):826–37.
58. Kobayashi T, Matsuyama T, Takeuchi M, et al. Autism spectrum disorder and prenatal exposure to selective serotonin reuptake inhibitors: a systematic review and meta-analysis. Reprod Toxicol 2016;65:170–8.
59. Ross LE, Grigoriadis S, Mamisashvili L, et al. Selected pregnancy and delivery outcomes after exposure to antidepressant medication: a systematic review and meta-analysis. JAMA Psychiatry 2013;70(4):436–43.
60. Hemels ME, Einarson A, Koren G, et al. Antidepressant use during pregnancy and the rates of spontaneous abortions: a meta-analysis. Ann Pharmacother 2005;39(5):803–9.
61. Nakhai-Pour HR, Broy P, Berard A. Use of antidepressants during pregnancy and the risk of spontaneous abortion. CMAJ 2010;182(10):1031–7.
62. Pearlstein T. Use of psychotropic medication during pregnancy and the postpartum period. Womens Health (Lond) 2013;9(6):605–15.
63. Webster PA. Withdrawal symptoms in neonates associated with maternal antidepressant therapy. Lancet 1973;2(7824):318–9.
64. Moses-Kolko EL, Bogen D, Perel J, et al. Neonatal signs after late in utero exposure to serotonin reuptake inhibitors: literature review and implications for clinical applications. JAMA 2005;293(19):2372–83.
65. Oberlander TF, Misri S, Fitzgerald CE, et al. Pharmacologic factors associated with transient neonatal symptoms following prenatal psychotropic medication exposure. J Clin Psychiatry 2004;65(2):230–7.
66. Moretti ME. Psychotropic drugs in lactation–Motherisk Update 2008. Can J Clin Pharmacol 2009;16(1):e49–57.
67. Bromley RL, Mawer GE, Briggs M, et al. The prevalence of neurodevelopmental disorders in children prenatally exposed to antiepileptic drugs. J Neurol Neurosurg Psychiatry 2013;84(6):637–43.
68. Christensen J, Gronborg TK, Sorensen MJ, et al. Prenatal valproate exposure and risk of autism spectrum disorders and childhood autism. JAMA 2013; 309(16):1696–703.
69. Cunnington M, Tennis P. Lamotrigine and the risk of malformations in pregnancy. Neurology 2005;64(6):955–60.
70. Holmes LB, Baldwin EJ, Smith CR, et al. Increased frequency of isolated cleft palate in infants exposed to lamotrigine during pregnancy. Neurology 2008; 70(22 Pt 2):2152–8.
71. Dolk H, Jentink J, Loane M, et al. Does lamotrigine use in pregnancy increase orofacial cleft risk relative to other malformations? Neurology 2008;71(10): 714–22.
72. Clark CT, Klein AM, Perel JM, et al. Lamotrigine dosing for pregnant patients with bipolar disorder. Am J Psychiatry 2013;170(11):1240–7.
73. Cohen LS, Friedman JM, Jefferson JW, et al. A reevaluation of risk of in utero exposure to lithium. JAMA 1994;271(2):146–50.

74. Jacobson SJ, Jones K, Johnson K, et al. Prospective multicentre study of pregnancy outcome after lithium exposure during first trimester. Lancet 1992; 339(8792):530–3.
75. Bogen DL, Sit D, Genovese A, et al. Three cases of lithium exposure and exclusive breastfeeding. Arch Womens Ment Health 2012;15(1):69–72.
76. Robinson GE. Treatment of schizophrenia in pregnancy and postpartum. J Popul Ther Clin Pharmacol 2012;19(3):e380–6.
77. Vigod SN, Gomes T, Wilton AS, et al. Antipsychotic drug use in pregnancy: high dimensional, propensity matched, population based cohort study. BMJ 2015; 350:h2298.
78. Newport DJ, Calamaras MR, DeVane CL, et al. Atypical antipsychotic administration during late pregnancy: placental passage and obstetrical outcomes. Am J Psychiatry 2007;164(8):1214–20.
79. Seeman MV. Clinical interventions for women with schizophrenia: pregnancy. Acta Psychiatr Scand 2013;127(1):12–22.
80. Newham JJ, Thomas SH, MacRitchie K, et al. Birth weight of infants after maternal exposure to typical and atypical antipsychotics: prospective comparison study. Br J Psychiatry 2008;192(5):333–7.
81. Paton C. Prescribing in pregnancy. Br J Psychiatry 2008;192(5):321–2.
82. Gentile S. Clinical utilization of atypical antipsychotics in pregnancy and lactation. Ann Pharmacother 2004;38(7–8):1265–71.
83. Khalifeh H, Dolman C, Howard LM. Safety of psychotropic drugs in pregnancy. BMJ 2015;350:h2260.
84. Gentile S. Antipsychotic therapy during early and late pregnancy. A systematic review. Schizophr Bull 2010;36(3):518–44.
85. Coppola D, Russo LJ, Kwarta RF Jr, et al. Evaluating the postmarketing experience of risperidone use during pregnancy: pregnancy and neonatal outcomes. Drug Saf 2007;30(3):247–64.
86. Communication FDS. Antipsychotic drug labels updated on use during pregnancy and risk of abnormal muscle movements and withdrawal symptoms in newborns. 2011. Available at: http://www.fda.gov/Drugs/DrugSafety/ucm243903.htm - sa. Accessed April 28, 2015.
87. Barnes TR. Evidence-based guidelines for the pharmacological treatment of schizophrenia: recommendations from the British Association for Psychopharmacology. J Psychopharmacol 2011;25(5):567–620.
88. Altshuler LL, Cohen L, Szuba MP, et al. Pharmacologic management of psychiatric illness during pregnancy: dilemmas and guidelines. Am J Psychiatry 1996; 153(5):592–606.
89. Thiels C. Pharmacotherapy of psychiatric disorder in pregnancy and during breastfeeding: a review. Pharmacopsychiatry 1987;20(4):133–46.
90. Peng M, Gao K, Ding Y, et al. Effects of prenatal exposure to atypical antipsychotics on postnatal development and growth of infants: a case-controlled, prospective study. Psychopharmacology (Berl) 2013;228(4):577–84.
91. Johnson KC, LaPrairie JL, Brennan PA, et al. Prenatal antipsychotic exposure and neuromotor performance during infancy. Arch Gen Psychiatry 2012;69(8): 787–94.
92. Iqbal MM, Sobhan T, Ryals T. Effects of commonly used benzodiazepines on the fetus, the neonate, and the nursing infant. Psychiatr Serv 2002;53(1):39–49.
93. Lin AE, Peller AJ, Westgate MN, et al. Clonazepam use in pregnancy and the risk of malformations. Birth Defects Res A Clin Mol Teratol 2004;70(8):534–6.

94. Oberlander TF, Gingrich JA, Ansorge MS. Sustained neurobehavioral effects of exposure to SSRI antidepressants during development: molecular to clinical evidence. Clin Pharmacol Ther 2009;86(6):672–7.
95. Holmes LB, Hernandez-Diaz S. Newer anticonvulsants: lamotrigine, topiramate and gabapentin. Birth Defects Res A Clin Mol Teratol 2012;94(8):599–606.
96. Molgaard-Nielsen D, Hviid A. Newer-generation antiepileptic drugs and the risk of major birth defects. JAMA 2011;305(19):1996–2002.
97. Fujii H, Goel A, Bernard N, et al. Pregnancy outcomes following gabapentin use: results of a prospective comparative cohort study. Neurology 2013;80(17): 1565–70.
98. Pottegard A, Hallas J, Andersen JT, et al. First-trimester exposure to methylphenidate: a population-based cohort study. J Clin Psychiatry 2014;75(1):e88–93.
99. Bro SP, Kjaersgaard MI, Parner ET, et al. Adverse pregnancy outcomes after exposure to methylphenidate or atomoxetine during pregnancy. Clin Epidemiol 2015;7:139–47.
100. Haervig KB, Mortensen LH, Hansen AV, et al. Use of ADHD medication during pregnancy from 1999 to 2010: a Danish register-based study. Pharmacoepidemiol Drug Saf 2014;23(5):526–33.

Depression and Menopause

An Update on Current Knowledge and Clinical Management for this Critical Window

Claudio N. Soares, MD, PhD, FRCPC, MBA[a,b,*]

KEYWORDS

- Depression • Menopause • Hot flashes • Anxiety • Sleep
- Estrogen therapy and mood regulation • Nonhormonal interventions

KEY POINTS

- Depression is a disabling condition, which often leads to significant personal, societal, and economic costs.
- Windows of vulnerability for depression likely are associated with an increased sensitivity to changes in the hormonal milieu experienced by some (but not all) women during the luteal phase of their cycles, the postpartum period, and/or during the menopause transition.
- An increased awareness of those windows of vulnerability has resulted in greater adoption of screening tools for mood and behavioral changes and tailored therapies for postpartum-related depressive episodes.
- Therapies uniquely designed for menopause-related depression are still debated. Part of the controversy has derived from conflicting methodologies to characterize reproductive staging or assess psychiatric conditions, and different targeted populations identified and assessed for the efficacy and tolerability of various antidepressant treatments, hormone therapies, or other interventions.

INTRODUCTION

Depression is a disabling condition that affects more than 300 million people worldwide and often leads to significant personal, societal, and economic costs. It affects 1 in every 5 adults in North America, with women being disproportionately more

This is an update of an article that first appeared in the *Psychiatric Clinics of North America*, Volume 40, Issue 2, June 2017.
Disclosure: Dr C.N. Soares has received research and educational grants from the Ontario Brain Institute (OBI) and the Ontario Research Funds–Research Excellence (ORF-RE). He has served as a consultant for Pfizer, Sunovion, Merck, Otsuka, Servier, and Lundbeck.
[a] Department of Psychiatry, Queen's University School of Medicine, 752 King Street West, Kingston, Ontario K7L 4X3, Canada; [b] Research and Innovation, Providence Care Hospital, Kingston, Ontario, Canada
* Department of Psychiatry, Queen's University School of Medicine, 752 King Street West, Kingston, Ontario K7L 4X3, Canada.
E-mail address: c.soares@queensu.ca

Med Clin N Am 103 (2019) 651–667
https://doi.org/10.1016/j.mcna.2019.03.001 medical.theclinics.com

affected than men. Such an increased risk (2-fold on average) has been the subject of debate and research over the years and from different viewpoints, including epidemiology, genetics, socioeconomic determinants of health, coping strategies, and hormone variations.[1,2]

Several researchers have been instrumental in proposing a paradigm to examine why some (but not all) women would be more likely to experience greater vulnerability for depression at certain stages (or windows) across the lifespan.[3–7] Based on this paradigm, the notion of windows of vulnerability for depression, also known as reproductive-related depressive episodes, was postulated to describe an increased sensitivity experienced by some women to changes in the hormonal milieu that occur during the luteal phase of their cycles, during the postpartum period, and/or during the menopause transition.

There has been an increased awareness of those windows of vulnerability, which is reflected in greater adoption of screening tools for mood and behavioral changes in the postpartum period, as well as the recognition by the American Psychiatric Association of the severity and functional impairment associated with the occurrence of premenstrual dysphoric disorder (PMDD). This has led to the inclusion of PMDD as a diagnostic category in the *Diagnostic and Statistical Manual of Mental Disorders, 5th edition*. Likewise, researchers and clinicians have developed therapeutic strategies tailored to reproductive-related mood events such as postpartum depression.[8]

The existence of a menopause-associated depression has been a more controversial point, despite undeniable evidence that this stage in life might be accompanied by other medical conditions, cardiovascular issues, vasomotor symptoms, sleep problems, and stressful life events, just to name a few.[9] The controversy has been fueled by conflicting methodologies used to characterize reproductive staging or assess psychiatric conditions in various studies, and by the scarcity of trials in which this targeted population (midlife women with depression and well-characterized menopause staging) was properly ascertained and assessed for the efficacy and tolerability of various antidepressant treatments, hormone therapies, or other interventions.

Depression and Menopause: Some Facts and Guiding Principles

The heightened burden associated with a major depressive disorder (MDD) is undeniable at any given point in the life cycle. However, the occurrence and persistence of depressive symptoms (not fully meeting criteria for clinical depression) may also lead to psychosocial impairment and adversely affect overall health.[10,11] Therefore, it is important that clinicians keep a closer monitoring and periodically reassess the need for therapies to address bothersome depressive symptoms (eg, low mood, reduced motivation and enjoyment with usual activities, disrupted sleep) through the use of pharmacologic agents, behavioral or lifestyle changes, or other treatments.

Cross-sectional and prospective studies have now investigated a potential association between menopause staging and the risks for depressive symptoms or MDD (new onset or recurrent).[12] Overall, data from cross-sectional studies indicate that depressive symptoms might be endorsed by up to 70% of women during perimenopause compared with around 30% in premenopausal years. Longitudinal studies, perhaps representing a better strategy for the assessment of this potential association, have suggested an increased risk of 1.5-fold to 3.0-fold for the occurrence of depressive symptoms during the menopause transition.[13,14] Importantly, such increased risk was identified even among women with no previous episodes; that is, new onset of symptoms. Finally, cohort studies have documented an increased risk for clinical depression (MDD, 2-fold to 4-fold increased risk) throughout the menopause transition and early postmenopausal years.

Risk factors for depression associated with the menopausal years can be grouped into 2 categories:

1. Continuum of risk factors: Longitudinal studies have identified risk factors for the occurrence of midlife depression that seem pervasive throughout the lifespan; these constitute a continuum of risk for depression and most likely act as moderating factors. These factors could be characterized as demographic or socioeconomic (ie, unemployment, low education, being black or Hispanic), health-related (eg, greater body mass index, being a smoker, reporting poor health and impaired functioning due to chronic medical conditions), and psychosocial (eg, poor social support, history of anxiety, 1 or more stressful life events). Importantly, a previous depressive episode is the strongest predictor for depression during midlife years, whereas a history of mood symptoms with a hormone-related context (ie, history of premenstrual syndrome, PMDD, or postpartum depression) has been moderately linked to depressive symptoms during the menopause transition and early postmenopausal years.
2. Window of risk–related factors: Researchers have also investigated the role of timing-related, context-related factors. Again, data from cross-sectional and longitudinal studies were valuable sources and helped identify mediating or precipitating factors associated with menopause-related depression. These factors include hormone variations (ie, the experience of wider fluctuations in follicle-stimulating hormone [FSH] and estradiol [E2] levels over time), menopause-related symptoms (eg, the presence and severity of vasomotor symptoms, sleep problems), overall health (current poor health, low functioning due to chronic medical conditions), and psychosocial stressors (including poor social support and stressful life events). The latter is characterized not only by the magnitude and number of events but also based on the temporal proximity (ie, timing of their occurrence in relation to the menopause transition per se).

Long-term trajectories

More recent studies have taken a closer look at prospective data to determine mediators for distinct trajectories of depressive symptoms throughout the menopause transition and beyond. The Study of Women's Health Across the Nation (SWAN) used data from a 13-year follow-up period to examine the course of clinical depression. The SWAN investigators determined that about 30% of those who developed depression at some point during the study ultimately experienced evolution into a persistent or recurrent condition. This was true even among those with new-onset cases of depression. Sleep problems and recent upsetting life events were among contributing factors to more persistent and/or recurrent depressive outcomes.[15,16] The Australian Longitudinal Study on Women's Health, on the other hand, identified 4 distinct patterns for depressive symptoms over a 15-year follow-up based on changes in the Center for Epidemiologic Studies Depression Scale (CES-D) scores over time: stable low (80.0%), increasing scores (9.0%), decreasing scores (8.5%), and stable high (2.5%). Those exhibiting stable high or increasing depressive symptoms over time (around 10%) were likely to experience continuum of risk factors such as previous diagnosis or treatment of depression and socioeconomic challenges. There were also context-related risk factors such as the exposure to a prolonged perimenopause or a surgically induced menopause.[17]

The role of anxiety and sleep

Anxiety and sleep problems are often identified as contributing factors to greater psychiatric morbidity among midlife women. Anxiety disorders constitute a heterogeneous group in which comorbid conditions are quite common and symptoms may overlap considerably. SWAN investigators attempted to explore 4 components or symptoms of anxiety (irritability, nervousness or tension, feeling fearful for no reason, and heart pounding or racing) and categorized their occurrence as high or low anxiety based on their scoring on the General Anxiety Disorder-7 scale.[18] They also examined whether anxiety symptoms at study entry would be more likely or less likely to occur during or after the menopausal transition than in their premenopausal years, regardless of the presence of vasomotor symptoms, health factors, or psychosocial stressors. Overall, women with high anxiety symptoms at study entry maintained significant rates of anxiety (16%–21%) throughout the 10-year follow-up period. Interestingly, the percentage of documented high anxiety visits declined from 71.4% (occurring during premenopausal years) to 30.0% (in the postmenopausal period). Moreover, those who reported high anxiety at baseline experienced a peak in symptoms during late perimenopausal years (13.5%), which is a much higher percentage than those observed in premenopausal years (4.6%), suggesting a possible window of vulnerability for increased anxiety in some women during midlife years.

More recently, Freeman and Sammel[19] (2016) examined the association between anxiety and severity of hot flashes over a 14-year follow-up interval (Penn Ovarian Aging Cohort). Somatic anxiety was strongly associated with hot flashes in the menopause transition, even after adjusting for important factors such as age, menopausal staging, reproductive hormone levels, history of depression, and others. Importantly, rather than cooccurring with vasomotor symptoms, somatic anxiety actually predicted the risk of further developing moderate or severe hot flashes.

Clinicians and patients often question whether sleep problems in midlife years represent a primary condition or an expression of an underlying problem (eg, presence of vasomotor symptoms or depression). Kravitz and colleagues[20] investigated possible interactions between menopause changes and sleep, and found an association between changes in bleeding patterns during the menopause transition and the emergence of sleep disturbances. Others indicated that women experiencing depression and vasomotor symptoms are likely to report poorer perceived sleep quality despite the lack of objective measures of sleep disruption; that is, an actual increase in number of awakenings or night sweats, or even significant changes in wakefulness after sleep onset (WASO) time.[21,22]

Joffe and colleagues[23] submitted 39 healthy, premenopausal women to gonadal hormone suppression by administering leuprolide to examine the independent contribution of hot flashes and sleep disturbances to the emergence of depressive symptoms among estrogen-deprived women. After 4 weeks of leuprolide use, 20 women (69%) developed hot flushes, whereas only 1 subject developed clinical depression. The increase in depressive symptoms (Montgomery-Åsberg Depression Rating Scale [MADRS] scores) was associated with objective and subjective changes in sleep patterns. However, only nocturnal hot flashes (and not daytime vasomotor symptoms) seemed to be significantly associated with an increase in depressive symptoms, even after adjusting for changes on sleep, suggesting that disturbed sleep does not fully explain the association of nocturnal hot flashes and mood disturbance in women experiencing estrogen depletion due to surgical or natural menopause.

Lampio and colleagues[24] (2016) examined the effects of aging and menopausal hormonal changes on sleep architecture during the menopause transition (6-year follow-up). The investigators collected overnight polysomnography recordings at baseline and at the follow-up visit, as well as FSH levels over time. Both aging and increased FSH concentration had an impact on sleep architecture. The age-related changes included shorter total sleep time, lower sleep efficiency, and greater sleep fragmentation; for example, increased WASO. Clinical characteristics and increased FSH levels (a marker of transition from premenopause to postmenopause) were associated with higher proportion of slow wave sleep and increased WASO.

WHAT ABOUT THE ESTROGEN CONNECTION?

Estrogen and Mood Regulation

The mediating effects of estrogen on monoaminergic systems, namely serotonin (5-hydroxytryptamine [5-HT]) and noradrenaline (NE) neurotransmission, may contribute to the development of depressive symptoms in women.[25–27] The presence and wide distribution of estrogen receptors in the brain and the estrogen activity found in regions known to be involved in mood and cognitive regulation (eg, prefrontal cortex, hippocampus) are contributing arguments to the notion that estrogen exerts mediating effects (and possibly therapeutic effects) on mood.[25,28,29]

Overall, the effects of E on 5-HT and NE could be characterized as beneficial to mood.[30] E2 administration limits the activity of monoamine oxidases (MAOs) A and B, which are enzymes involved in 5-HT degradation.[31] It also increases both isoforms of tryptophan hydroxylase, the rate-limiting enzyme of serotonin synthesis.[32,33] Thus, E2 administration results in an overall net increase in 5-HT synthesis and availability. Moreover, estrogens increased 5-HT receptor density in brain regions containing E receptors, such as the hypothalamus, the preoptic area, and the amygdala.[34–37] E2 downregulates $5HT_{1a}$ auto-receptors and upregulates $5HT_{2a}$ receptors, increasing the amount of serotonin found in the synapse and consequently the amount available for postsynaptic transmission. Estrogen effects also promote NE availability by decreasing the expression of MAOs and increasing the activity of tyrosine hydroxylase, the rate-limiting enzyme in the synthesis of catecholamine.[38,39] Acute E2 administration increases dopamine β-hydroxylase (DBH) gene transcription; DBH catalyzes the hydroxylation of dopamine to form NE. In sum, estrogen works via distinct pathways to regulate synthesis, metabolism, and receptor density or activity of the classical neurotransmitters implicated in mood regulation.[40,41] Finally, estrogen may also have mood-enhancing (or antidepressant-like) properties due to its stimulating effect on brain-derived neurotrophic factor, an important neuroprotective agent at multiple levels.[42]

Estrogen Therapy for Depression: Level I Evidence of a Critical Window

Despite some evidence of E2 antidepressant properties, particularly among depressed, perimenopausal women, the acceptability of estrogen therapy (ET) as part of the therapeutic armamentarium for depression remains limited. A recent, comprehensive systematic review examined the efficacy of estrogen-based interventions for depression.[30] Potentially relevant studies were selected based on the following criteria: (1) clinical administration of estrogen-based, hormone therapy and (2) assessment of mood symptoms or depression with standardized instruments.

Surprisingly, only a few randomized controlled trials (RCTs) have examined the benefits of ET on clinically depressed women. Most studies included women who were either asymptomatic or mildly affected at study entry, again making it more difficult to generalize and/or compare their findings. Thus, given the scarce number of RCTs with estrogen-based therapies for menopause depression, the author has expanded the review conducted by Rubinow and colleagues and included open-label, single-blind, and double-blind interventions.

The author also recognizes that clinical trials have not been the only source of information for a better understanding of the effects of estrogen on mood. Some have explored the brain-related effects of estrogen in longitudinal observational studies; for example, by comparing women who underwent oophorectomy before the onset of menopause (average follow-up 25 years) to an aged-matched sample from the same community; a particular study demonstrated that those who underwent surgery had a significant increased risk for developing depressive and anxiety symptoms when compared with the referent group.[43] The risks were even greater among those who underwent surgery at younger age, leading the author to speculate a potential association of these findings with an early loss of neuroprotective effects of estrogen during reproductive years.

Mood Regulation: Estrogen Therapies in Nondepressed Women

Perimenopausal women

A single RCT assessed mood in strictly nondepressed, perimenopausal women (N = 83, aged 40–52 years).[44] Menopausal staging was based on menstrual patterns and the presence of vasomotor symptoms, whereas depressive symptoms were assessed via a standardized instrument: the Zung Self Rating Depression Scale. This was a 6-month, crossover study comparing a hormone treatment (estrogen-progestin therapy [EPT]) with 2 weeks of conjugated equine estrogen (CEE) followed by 2 weeks of CEE plus medroxyprogesterone acetate (MPA). No significant effects on mood were observed when the order of treatment allocation was ignored. Study limitations included the lack of a calibration or run-in period, and the treatment duration.

In a recent pilot study of perimenopausal women (N = 38, aged 38–52 years) who were predominantly nondepressed, the investigators compared the effects of levonorgestrel-containing intrauterine system (LNG-IUS) plus low-dose transdermal E2 (gel 0.06% containing 0.75 mg E2 per 1.25 g metered dose) to LNG-IUS alone (plus inactive gel) for 50 days. The study assessed depressive symptoms using the CES-D, the impact of hot flashes using the Hot Flash–Related Daily Interference Scale, fatigue using the Fatigue Severity Scale, and sleep characteristics via the Pittsburgh Sleep Quality Index. Although most women were symptomatic with respect to hot flashes (61%) and poor sleep (71%), only a small number reported significant depressive symptoms (CES-D scores >16, n = 5 or 13%) or fatigue (n = 5, 13%) at study entry. Overall, the study revealed beneficial effects of LNG-IUS plus TDE for the improvement of hot flashes and daytime fatigue, with minimal or nonsignificant effects on sleep and no significant changes in mood (improvement or worsening).[45]

To date, only 1 randomized trial has investigated the efficacy of estrogen in preventing the onset of significant depressive symptoms in perimenopausal and early postmenopausal women. Euthymic perimenopausal or early postmenopausal women (n = 172) were assigned to receive either transdermal E2 (0.1 mg/d) plus intermittent oral micronized progesterone (200 mg/d for 12 days every 3 months) or placebo patches plus pills. After 12 months, women receiving active HT were significantly less likely to develop depressive symptoms compared with women receiving placebo (32.3% vs 17.3%). Those in the early perimenopausal stage (but not late perimenopausal or early postmenopausal stages) benefited the most from estrogen as a preventive strategy. The benefits were also modified by stressful life events, with greater benefits for women who had experienced stressful life events in the preceding 6 months of the intervention. Vasomotor symptoms and prior history of MDD did not modify the effect of HT on depressive symptoms. These findings, if further replicated, highlight the importance of a careful clinical interview to facilitate personalized interventions for midlife women.

Postmenopausal women

The effects of HT on mood have been assessed in clinical studies in younger, postmenopausal women (ie, up to 10 years postmenopause and aged <70 years). In most studies, the presence of menopause-related symptoms (ie, vasomotor, sleep, pain) was documented at study entry, making the alleviation of these symptoms with hormone interventions an important factor (mediating and/or confounding) to be considered. Haines and colleagues[46] (2003) studied 152 postmenopausal women (posthysterectomy, aged 48 $\pm$ 5 years) in a randomized, double-blind placebo-controlled trial of 1 or 2 mg of oral E2 or placebo for 12 months (primary outcome: prevention of bone loss, ie, reduced risk for osteoporosis). Women had their depressive symptoms assessed via the Hospital Anxiety and Depression Scale and their psychological wellbeing and quality of life (QOL) using the World Health Organization QOL questionnaire. Over a 12-month follow-up period, menopausal symptoms were significantly reduced in the 2 mg arm (not among those using 1 mg or placebo), whereas no significant changes in mood or QOL were observed (from mild or no significant impairment observed at baseline).

Fifty-four asymptomatic postmenopausal women (average age 52 $\pm$ 4 years) were randomized to receive oral ET (CEE 0.625 mg/d), EPT (CEE + MPA, 10 mg/d), or placebo in a 6-month trial. Subjects were recruited based on the absence of psychiatric symptoms (HAM-D and HAM-A scales) and assessed at baseline and endpoint for psychological symptoms using the Beck Depression Inventory (BDI) and the Profile of Moods States. Hormone treatment did not lead to a significant change in mood over time when compared with placebo.[47]

In another trial (3-month duration), 183 postmenopausal women (average age 48 years, postmenopausal for at least 1 year) were recruited based on the presence of severe menopausal symptoms and randomized into 3 treatment groups: (1) transdermal E2 plus oral norethisterone acetate, (2) oral continuous combination of norethisterone and E2 hemihydrate, or (3) placebo. Menopausal, depressive, and anxiety symptoms were assessed using the Kupperman scale, the Hamilton Depression Rating Scale (HDRS), and the Beck Anxiety Inventory (BAI), respectively. Compared with placebo, the use of transdermal E2 (alone or in combination with norethisterone) led to a significant improvement of menopausal symptoms, as well as reduction in HDRS and BAI scores depression and anxiety symptoms.[48]

Almeida and colleagues[49] examined the benefits of ET (oral E2, 2 mg/d) for cognition, mood, and QOL in older postmenopausal women (n = 115, average age 73 years) in a 20-week randomized double-blind placebo-controlled trial. Outcome measures included changes in the BDI, changes in QOL scores (SF-36), and cognitive function (CAMCOG, Block Design, Memory for Faces, California Verbal Learning Test, and verbal fluency). After 20 weeks of treatment, unopposed estrogen administered orally was not associated with significant changes in cognitive function, mood, or QOL.

In another placebo-controlled trial, 412 postmenopausal women (average age 71 years) were allocated into 4 different treatment groups: ET with 0.625 of CEE, CEE plus 2.5 mg of MPA, calcitriol 0.25 g twice a day alone, and a combination of HT and calcitriol. Depression symptoms were assessed via the Geriatric Depression Scale (GDS) at baseline and at the end of the 36-month trial. GDS scores suggested that about 12% of the sample was depressed at study entry. No significant effects of hormone treatment on mood were observed at endpoint, and the percentage of depressed women (based on GDS scores) decreased across all treatment groups.[50]

In sum, these results suggest a lack of significant beneficial effects of estrogen on mood (ie, mood improvement) when administered to nondepressed women, particularly in their postmenopausal years. Preliminary but promising results suggest a potential role for estrogen in mitigating the risk for developing depressive symptoms among specific at-risk subpopulations transitioning to menopause.

Additional information has been derived from large trials such as the Heart and Estrogen/Progestin Replacement Study (HERS),[51] the Women's Health Initiative Study of Cognitive Aging (WHISCA)[52,53] and the Women's International Study of long Duration Estrogen after the Menopause (WISDOM).[54,55] These studies offered additional opportunities to examine the effects of hormone therapies on mood and QOL among both younger and older nondepressed postmenopausal women. Altogether, these studies failed to demonstrate a significant impact of hormone therapies on mood and reiterate the notion that estrogen-based therapies should not be considered as a strategy for prevention or alleviation of mood symptoms in otherwise nondepressed, asymptomatic perimenopausal, or postmenopausal women.[30] Recent data from the Kronos Early Estrogen Prevention Study (KEEPS) examined the effects of estrogen-based therapies on mood symptoms among nondepressed, early postmenopausal women.[56,57] Contrary to other studies, the investigators identified a positive impact on mood with the use of oral CEEs but not with transdermal E2.

Mood Improvement: The Use of Estrogen Therapies in Depressed Women

Perimenopausal women

At least 4 small studies, including 2 RCTs, have demonstrated the efficacy of E2 for the management of depressive disorders during perimenopause.[58–61] The 2 RCTS (Soares and Schmidt) had similar designs and are considered of high quality due to the utilization of standardized tools to confirm the diagnosis of depression and the characterization of menopausal staging using FSH levels and history of menstrual irregularity. In addition, treatment compliance was monitored by serum E2 measurements in both studies. Antidepressant effects were well-documented (reduction in CES-D, HDRS, and MADRS scores) and significant mood improvement was observed among those suffering from new-onset or recurrent MDD in the presence or absence of concomitant vasomotor symptoms. Moreover, the antidepressant effects of E2 persisted after a 4-week washout period, even after reemergence of hot flashes and night sweats.[61]

Estrogen has also been used as an augmentation strategy for women with unsatisfactory response to antidepressants. Most studies suggest that estrogen might augment clinical response to antidepressants, including selective serotonin reuptake inhibitors (SSRIs) and serotonin-norepinephrine reuptake inhibitor (SNRIs).[62–68]

Postmenopausal women

Two RCTs have assessed the use of hormone therapy in postmenopausal women with depressive disorders. Morrison and colleagues (2004) examined the efficacy of transdermal E2 (0.1 mg) compared with placebo in late postmenopausal women (N = 57; average age 67 years, postmenopausal for about 16 years) suffering from mild-to-moderate depression. After 8 weeks of treatment, both groups showed similar decrease in depressive symptoms based on changes in HDRS scores or self-assessed CES-D scores from baseline. The study also suggested that a subgroup of depressed postmenopausal women (ie, those with a past history of major depression) could be particularly responsive to placebo.

In another RCT, Rudolph and colleagues (2004) examined the effects of oral HT (a continuous combination of E2 valerate 2 mg and dienogest 2 mg/d) in a 24-week trial of 129 postmenopausal women. In this study, women were considerably younger (average age 55 years) and the use of HT led to significant improvements in depressive scores (reduction in HDRS scores). These findings, however, should be examined with caution given the unusually high dropout rates observed among treatment users (33%) and placebo users (58%).

Finally, an RCT included 72 women with depression and was confirmed by the Structured Clinical Interview for Axis I Disorders of mild to moderate severity (ie, MADRS) scores of 15 to 31 at study entry. Women were perimenopausal and postmenopausal (mean age 51.1 $\pm$ 5.0 years), experiencing sleep disturbances (insomnia syndrome) that affected their functioning and reporting 3 or more nights per week with significant hot flashes. Subjects were randomly assigned to transdermal 17β-E2 0.05 mg/d, zolpidem 10 mg/d, or placebo for 8 weeks. All groups showed improvement in depressive symptoms (MADRS scores); that is, the study failed to demonstrate meaningful differences between active treatment groups and placebo. Interestingly, overall improvement in mood was significantly correlated with an increase in serum E2 over time and improvement in perceived quality. It is plausible that an increase in E2 levels occurred due to ET use in 1 treatment arm and/or to naturally occurring fluctuations among study participants. Mood improvement, however, was not significantly correlated with suppression of hot flashes or changes in objectively measures of sleep.[69]

Schmidt and colleagues[70] tested the estrogen withdrawal theory (previously examined in premenstrual and postnatal populations) in asymptomatic postmenopausal women (N = 56) with history of perimenopausal depression. After 3 weeks of open-label administration of transdermal E2 (100 μg/d), study participants were randomized to receive either E2 or matched placebo skin patches for 3 additional weeks in a double-blind fashion. There were no reports of depressive symptoms during the open-label phase with E2. Women with history of perimenopausal depression who were crossed over from E2 to placebo reported an increase in depressive symptoms (assessed by the CES-D and HDRS), whereas those (also with past history of perimenopausal depression) who remained on E2 therapy continued to be asymptomatic. Of note, both groups had similar hot-flush severity and plasma E2 levels while on placebo. The study by Schmidt and colleagues[70] elegantly demonstrated that some midlife women could be particularly susceptible to developing behavioral or mood changes when exposed to changes in estrogen levels or secretion. These findings corroborate the notion of a critical timing to consider estrogen's role as a contributing and/or mitigating factor for depression in midlife women.

In sum, ET, particularly transdermal E2, has shown antidepressant effects of similar magnitude to that observed with classic antidepressant agents when administered to perimenopausal women suffering from clinical depression, whereas it seems to be ineffective as a mood enhancer among depression-free (asymptomatic) women. Transdermal 17β-E2 seems to lead to a greater antidepressant effect size (ie, drug-placebo difference) and could therefore constitute a potential treatment of depressed mood in this population.[71,72] On the other hand, the same hormone intervention formulation (E2) and route of administration (transdermally) was not effective in treating depressed postmenopausal women.[73,74] This particular finding suggests that the menopausal transition might not only be a critical window of risk for depression but also a window of opportunity for the effective use of estrogen therapies for depression in midlife years.[9] However, existing data on estrogen-based therapies for depressed perimenopausal and postmenopausal women are limited in terms of number of randomized trials, sample sizes recruited, and number of study completers (**Table 1**), making the interpretation and generalization or applicability of some of these findings more challenging.

Table 1
Randomized trials on estrogen therapies for symptomatic or depressed perimenopausal and postmenopausal women

Authors	Population Studied (Type, n)	Design	Intervention	Outcome Measures	Key Findings
Schmidt et al,[60] 2001	Perimenopause-related depression (n = 31)	DB, PL Parallel study followed by crossover, PL-controlled	ET (transdermal E2), followed by MPA	HDRS, CES-D scores	ET led to significant improvements in depressive symptoms (HDRS and CES-D scores)
Soares et al,[61] 2001	Perimenopause-related depression (n = 45)	DB, PL Parallel study	ET (transdermal E2)	MADRS scores	ET led to significant improvements in depressive symptoms (MADRS scores)
Rudolph et al,[75] 2004; Santoro,[76] 2005	Postmenopausal women with mild or moderate depressive symptoms (n = 129)	DB, PL Parallel study	EPT (oral E2 valerate + progestin [dienogest])	HDRS scores	EPT led to improvements in HDRS scores; high attrition rates in both groups
Morrison et al,[73] 2004	Postmenopausal women with depressive disorders (n = 57)	DB, PL Parallel study	ET (transdermal E2) followed by MPA	HDRS, CES-D scores	No differences with active treatment (both groups showed improvement)
Joffe et al,[69] 2011	Mixed perimenopausal and postmenopausal women with depressive symptoms, VMS and insomnia (n = 72)	DB, PL Parallel study	ET (transdermal E2), Zolpidem	MADRS, BDI, PSQI scores	No significant differences with respect to mood changes between treatment and PL groups

Abbreviations: DB, double-blind; PL, placebo; PSQI, Pittsburgh Sleep Quality Index.

FINAL CONSIDERATIONS AND RECOMMENDATIONS REGARDING ESTROGEN THERAPIES

There are indicators of windows of vulnerability for cardiovascular, mood, and cognitive conditions in midlife women; at the same time, the critical window hypothesis suggests the existence of a window of opportunity for the administration of E2 to symptomatic women across different systems or domains. Further investigation is needed to disentangle common underlying mechanisms.[77]

Clinicians should always consider the various treatment strategies available and determine the extent to which they can be tailored to address the multiple symptom domains for each patient. For example, based on the author's review and accumulated clinical experience, an argument can be made that perimenopausal women presenting with significant, bothersome menopausal symptoms (significant VMS) and concurrent depressive symptoms could benefit from an initial, brief trial (2–4 weeks) with transdermal E2 as a monotherapy to determine the benefits and tolerability of hormone treatment for the alleviation of both mood and menopausal symptoms. After that, the need for antidepressant use (monotherapy or concomitant use) could be reassessed. Obviously, women who experienced multiple depressive episodes in the past (not necessarily hormone-related), and women presenting with severe depressive symptoms and/or expressing suicidal ideation should always be evaluated and treated with more intensive, widely used antidepressant strategies.

The type of hormone treatment and route of administration should be carefully considered if alleviation of depression is an important goal. Different HT formulations (eg, transdermal E2 vs oral conjugated estrogens, E alone vs estrogen plus progestin therapies) should take into consideration not only the risks or benefits for bone and cardiovascular health but also for cognitive and mood functioning. So far, the evidence for the use of transdermal E2 for depression is more robust and reinforced by its absorption process (no hepatic first-pass effects) and overall safety profile.

WHAT ABOUT NONHORMONAL INTERVENTIONS?

Antidepressants remain the first-line treatment of depression during midlife years, particularly for those who experienced multiple depressive episodes in the past (not necessarily hormone-related), reporting severe symptoms or significant functional impairment, and/or expressing suicidal ideation. For recurrent episodes, a previous response to a specific antidepressant (agent, class) should guide the primary decision on what to try first. For those experiencing depression for the first time, those who are treatment-naïve, or those presenting with history of partial or no response to antidepressants past, existing data support the efficacy and tolerability of various SSRIs and SNRIs at usual doses. There are studies on fluoxetine, sertraline, venlafaxine, citalopram, escitalopram, duloxetine, desvenlafaxine, and vortioxetine.[78–86]

Existing data do not support superior efficacy of a particular antidepressant agent or class over the others for the management of midlife depression. Still, a few important points should be taken into consideration when choosing an antidepressant for this population. First, despite small numbers and methodological limitations, data on efficacy and tolerability of various agents for this particular population could inform and guide some of the preliminary discussions with midlife women suffering from depression. Second, data on tolerability and adverse events (and how they seem to affect treatment adherence) should be carefully examined, particularly when issues such as sexual dysfunction and changes in metabolism are already part of the clinical scenario or reported as important concerns. Conversely, look for data supporting the efficacy of some of the antidepressants for the relief of menopause-related symptoms (eg, hot flashes, pain, disrupted sleep) and QOL improvement. Finally, data available on drug safety (eg, drug-drug interactions) should always be considered because multiple medications that are often prescribed to this population.[87]

SUMMARY

Evidence-based psychotherapies, particularly behavioral-based interventions, should have a place in the treatment armamentarium to ultimately reduce the overall burden and functional impairment associated with depression in this population.[88] Nonpharmacologic or hormonal strategies (eg, exercise, balanced diet, dietary supplements) need to be better examined as additional tools to help improve QOL and reduce functional impairment during the menopause transition and beyond.

REFERENCES

1. Steiner M. Female-specific mood disorders. Clin Obstet Gynecol 1992;35(3): 599–611.
2. Thurston RC, Joffe H, Soares CN, et al. Physical activity and risk of vasomotor symptoms in women with and without a history of depression: results from the Harvard Study of Moods and Cycles. Menopause 2006;13(4):553–60.
3. Bloch M, Schmidt PJ, Danaceau M, et al. Effects of gonadal steroids in women with a history of postpartum depression. Am J Psychiatry 2000;157(6):924–30.
4. Bloch M, Rotenberg N, Koren D, et al. Risk factors for early postpartum depressive symptoms. Gen Hosp Psychiatry 2006;28(1):3–8.
5. Boyle GJ, Murrihy R. A preliminary study of hormone replacement therapy and psychological mood states in perimenopausal women. Psychol Rep 2001; 88(1):160–70.
6. Bromberger JT, Harlow S, Avis N, et al. Racial/ethnic differences in the prevalence of depressive symptoms among middle-aged women: the Study of Women's Health Across the Nation (SWAN). Am J Public Health 2004;94(8): 1378–85.
7. Rubinow DR, Schmidt PJ, Roca CA. Estrogen-serotonin interactions: implications for affective regulation. Biol Psychiatry 1998;44(9):839–50.
8. Kanes S, Colquhoun H, Gunduz-Bruce H, et al. Brexanolone (SAGE-547 injection) in post-partum depression: a randomised controlled trial. Lancet 2017; 390(10093):480–9.
9. Soares CN. Mood disorders in midlife women: understanding the critical window and its clinical implications. Menopause 2014;21(2):198–206.
10. Pietrzak RH, Kinley J, Afifi TO, et al. Subsyndromal depression in the United States: prevalence, course, and risk for incident psychiatric outcomes. Psychol Med 2013;43(7):1401–14.
11. Rodríguez MR, Nuevo R, Chatterji S, et al. Definitions and factors associated with subthreshold depressive conditions: a systematic review. BMC Psychiatry 2012; 12:181.
12. Bromberger JT, Kravitz HM. Mood and menopause: findings from the Study of Women's Health Across the Nation (SWAN) over 10 years. Obstet Gynecol Clin North Am 2011;38(3):609–25.
13. Bromberger JT, Schott L, Kravitz HM, et al. Risk factors for major depression during midlife among a community sample of women with and without prior major depression: are they the same or different? Psychol Med 2015;45: 1653–64.

14. Freeman EW, Sammel MD, Lin H, et al. Associations of hormones and menopausal status with depressed mood in women with no history of depression. Arch Gen Psychiatry 2006;63:375–82.
15. Bromberger JT, Kravitz HM, Youk A, et al. Patterns of depressive disorders across 13 years and their determinants among midlife women: SWAN mental health study. J Affect Disord 2016;206:31–40.
16. Clayton AH, Pinkerton JV. Vulnerability to depression and cardiometabolic risk associated with early ovarian disruption. Menopause 2013;20(6):598–9.
17. Hickey M, Schoenaker DA, Joffe H, et al. Depressive symptoms across the menopause transition: findings from a large population-based cohort study. Menopause 2016;23(12):1287–93.
18. Bromberger JT, Kravitz HM, Chang Y, et al. Does risk for anxiety increase during the menopausal transition? Study of women's health across the nation. Menopause 2013;20(5):488–95.
19. Freeman EW, Sammel MD. Anxiety as a risk factor for menopausal hot flashes: evidence from the Penn Ovarian Aging cohort. Menopause 2016;23(9):942–9.
20. Kravitz HM, Zhao X, Bromberger JT, et al. Sleep disturbance during the menopausal transition in a multi-ethnic community sample of women. Sleep 2008; 31(7):979–90.
21. Joffe H, Soares CN, Thurston RC, et al. Depression is associated with worse objectively and subjectively measured sleep, but not more frequent awakenings, in women with vasomotor symptoms. Menopause 2009;16(4):671–9.
22. Joffe H, Massler A, Sharkey KM. Evaluation and management of sleep disturbance during the menopause transition. Semin Reprod Med 2010;28(5):404–21.
23. Joffe H, Crawford SL, Freeman MP, et al. Independent contributions of nocturnal hot flashes and sleep disturbance to depression in estrogen-deprived women. J Clin Endocrinol Metab 2016;101(10):3847–55.
24. Lampio L, Polo-Kantola P, Himanen SL, et al. Sleep during menopausal transition: a 6-year follow-up. Sleep 2017;40(7). https://doi.org/10.1093/sleep/zsx090.
25. McEwen BS, Alves SE. Estrogen actions in the central nervous system. Endocr Rev 1999;20(3):279–307.
26. Lokuge S, Frey BN, Foster JA, et al. Depression in women: windows of vulnerability and new insights into the link between estrogen and serotonin. J Clin Psychiatry 2011;72(11):e1563–9.
27. Yonkers KA, O'Brien PM, Eriksson E. Premenstrual syndrome. Lancet 2008; 371(9619):1200–10.
28. Deecher D, Andree TH, Sloan D, et al. From menarche to menopause: exploring the underlying biology of depression in women experiencing hormonal changes. Psychoneuroendocrinology 2008;33(1):3–17.
29. Genazzani AR, Bernardi F, Pluchino N, et al. Endocrinology of menopausal transition and its brain implications. CNS Spectr 2005;10(6):449–57.
30. Rubinow DR, Johnson SL, Schmidt PJ, et al. Efficacy of estradiol in perimenopausal depression: so much promise and so few answers. Depress Anxiety 2015;32(8):539–49.
31. Gundlah C, Lu NZ, Bethea CL. Ovarian steroid regulation of monoamine oxidase-A and -B mRNAs in the macaque dorsal raphe and hypothalamic nuclei. Psychopharmacology (Berl) 2002;160(3):271–82.
32. Bethea CL, Mirkes SJ, Su A, et al. Effects of oral estrogen, raloxifene and arzoxifene on gene expression in serotonin neurons of macaques. Psychoneuroendocrinology 2002;27(4):431–45.

33. Hiroi R, McDevitt RA, Neumaier JF. Estrogen selectively increases tryptophan hydroxylase-2 mRNA expression in distinct subregions of rat midbrain raphe nucleus: association between gene expression and anxiety behavior in the open field. Biol Psychiatry 2006;60(3):288–95.
34. Biegon A, Reches A, Snyder L, et al. Serotonergic and noradrenergic receptors in the rat brain: modulation by chronic exposure to ovarian hormones. Life Sci 1983; 32(17):2015–21.
35. Cyr M, Bosse R, Di Paolo T. Gonadal hormones modulate 5-hydroxytryptamine2A receptors: emphasis on the rat frontal cortex. Neuroscience 1998;83(3):829–36.
36. Moses-Kolko EL, Wisner KL, Price JC, et al. Serotonin 1A receptor reductions in postpartum depression: a positron emission tomography study. Fertil Steril 2008; 89(3):685–92.
37. Nelson HD. Menopause. Lancet 2008;371(9614):760–70.
38. Pau KY, Hess DL, Kohama S, et al. Oestrogen upregulates noradrenaline release in the mediobasal hypothalamus and tyrosine hydroxylase gene expression in the brainstem of ovariectomized rhesus macaques. J Neuroendocrinol 2000;12(9): 899–909.
39. Pérez-López FR, Pérez-Roncero G, Fernández-Iñarrea J, et al, MARIA (MenopAuse RIsk Assessment) Research Group. Resilience, depressed mood, and menopausal symptoms in postmenopausal women. Menopause 2014;21(2): 159–64.
40. Osterlund MK, Kuiper GG, Gustafsson JA, et al. Differential distribution and regulation of estrogen receptor-alpha and -beta mRNA within the female rat brain. Brain Res Mol Brain Res 1998;54(1):175–80.
41. Osterlund MK, Halldin C, Hurd YL. Effects of chronic 17beta-estradiol treatment on the serotonin 5-HT(1A) receptor mRNA and binding levels in the rat brain. Synapse 2000;35(1):39–44.
42. Srivastava DP, Woolfrey KM, Evans PD. Mechanisms underlying the interactions between rapid estrogenic and BDNF control of synaptic connectivity. Neuroscience 2013;239:17–33.
43. Rocca WA, Grossardt BR, Geda YE, et al. Long-term risk of depressive and anxiety symptoms after early bilateral oophorectomy. Menopause 2008;15(6): 1050–9.
44. Khoo SK, Coglan M, Battistutta D, et al. Hormonal treatment and psychological function during the menopausal transition: an evaluation of the effects of conjugated estrogens/cyclic medroxyprogesterone acetate. Climacteric 1998;1(1): 55–62.
45. Santoro N, Teal S, Gavito C, et al. Use of a levonorgestrel-containing intrauterine system with supplemental estrogen improves symptoms in perimenopausal women: a pilot study. Menopause 2015;22(12):1301–7.
46. Haines CJ, Yim SF, Chung TK, et al. A prospective, randomized, placebo-controlled study of the dose effect of oral oestradiol on menopausal symptoms, psychological well being, and quality of life in postmenopausal Chinese women. Maturitas 2003;44(3):207–14.
47. Girdler SS, O'Briant C, Steege J, et al. A comparison of the effect of estrogen with or without progesterone on mood and physical symptoms in postmenopausal women. J Womens Health Gend Based Med 1999;8(5):637–46.
48. Karsidag C, Karageyim Karsidag AY, Esim Buyukbayrak E, et al. Comparison of effects of two different hormone therapies on mood in symptomatic postmenopausal women. Archives of Neuropsychiatry 2012;49(1):39–43.

49. Almeida OP, Lautenschlager NT, Vasikaran S, et al. A 20-week randomized controlled trial of estradiol replacement therapy for women aged 70 years and older: effect on mood, cognition and quality of life. Neurobiol Aging 2006;27(1): 141–9.
50. Yalamanchili V, Gallagher JC. Treatment with hormone therapy and calcitriol did not affect depression in older postmenopausal women: no interaction with estrogen and vitamin D receptor genotype polymorphisms. Menopause 2012;19(6): 697–703.
51. Hlatky et al., 2002.
52. Resnick SM, Maki PM, Rapp SR, et al, Women's Health Initiative Study of Cognitive Aging Investigators. Effects of combination estrogen plus progestin hormone treatment on cognition and affect. J Clin Endocrinol Metab 2006;91(5):1802–10.
53. Resnick SM, Espeland MA, An Y, et al, Women's Health Initiative Study of Cognitive Aging Investigators. Effects of conjugated equine estrogens on cognition and affect in postmenopausal women with prior hysterectomy. J Clin Endocrinol Metab 2009;94(11):4152–61.
54. Welton AJ, Vickers MR, Kim J, et al, WISDOM team. Health related quality of life after combined hormone replacement therapy: randomised controlled trial. BMJ 2008;337:a1190.
55. Wittchen HU, Becker E, Lieb R, et al. Prevalence, incidence and stability of premenstrual dysphoric disorder in the community. Psychol Med 2002;32(1):119–32.
56. Gleason CE, Dowling NM, Wharton W, et al. Effects of hormone therapy on cognition and mood in recently postmenopausal women: findings from the randomized, controlled KEEPS-cognitive and affective study. PLoS Med 2015;12(6): e1001833.
57. Gordon JL, Rubinow DR, Eisenlohr-Moul TA, et al. Efficacy of transdermal estradiol and micronized progesterone in the prevention of depressive symptoms in the menopause transition: a randomized clinical trial. JAMA Psychiatry 2018; 75(2):149–57.
58. Cohen LS, Soares CN, Poitras JR, et al. Short-term use of estradiol for depression in perimenopausal and postmenopausal women: a preliminary report. Am J Psychiatry 2003;160(8):1519–22.
59. Rasgon NL, Altshuler LL, Fairbanks L. Estrogen-replacement therapy for depression. Am J Psychiatry 2001;158(10):1738.
60. Schmidt PJ, Nieman L, Danaceau MA, et al. Estrogen replacement in perimenopause-related depression: a preliminary report. Am J Obstet Gynecol 2000;183(2):414–20.
61. Soares CN, Almeida OP, Joffe H, et al. Efficacy of estradiol for the treatment of depressive disorders in perimenopausal women: a double-blind, randomized, placebo-controlled trial. Arch Gen Psychiatry 2001;58(6):529–34.
62. Amsterdam J, Garcia-Espana F, Fawcett J, et al. Fluoxetine efficacy in menopausal women with and without estrogen replacement. J Affect Disord 1999; 55(1):11–7.
63. Entsuah AR, Huang H, Thase ME. Response and remission rates in different subpopulations with major depressive disorder administered venlafaxine, selective serotonin reuptake inhibitors, or placebo. J Clin Psychiatry 2001;62(11):869–77.
64. Schneider LS, Small GW, Hamilton SH, et al. Estrogen replacement and response to fluoxetine in a multicenter geriatric depression trial. Fluoxetine Collaborative Study Group. Am J Geriatr Psychiatry 1997;5(2):97–106.

65. Schneider LS, Small GW, Clary CM. Estrogen replacement therapy and antidepressant response to sertraline in older depressed women. Am J Geriatr Psychiatry 2001;9(4):393–9.
66. Soares CN, Poitras JR, Prouty J, et al. Efficacy of citalopram as a monotherapy or as an adjunctive treatment to estrogen therapy for perimenopausal and postmenopausal women with depression and vasomotor symptoms. J Clin Psychiatry 2003;64(4):473–9.
67. Soares CN, Arsenio H, Joffe H, et al. Escitalopram versus ethinyl estradiol and norethindrone acetate for symptomatic peri- and postmenopausal women: impact on depression, vasomotor symptoms, sleep, and quality of life. Menopause 2006;13(5):780–6.
68. Soares CN. Menopausal transition and depression: who is at risk and how to treat it? Expert Rev Neurother 2007;7(10):1285–93.
69. Joffe H, Petrillo LF, Koukopoulos A, et al. Increased estradiol and improved sleep, but not hot flashes, predict enhanced mood during the menopausal transition. J Clin Endocrinol Metab 2011;96(7):E1044–54.
70. Schmidt PJ, Ben Dor R, Martinez PE, et al. Effects of estradiol withdrawal on mood in women with past perimenopausal depression: a randomized clinical trial. JAMA Psychiatry 2015;72(7):714–26.
71. Stahl S. Effects of estrogen on the central nervous system. J Clin Psychiatry 2001; 62(5):317–8.
72. Stahl SM. Vasomotor symptoms and depression in women, part I. Role of vasomotor symptoms in signaling the onset or relapse of a major depressive episode. J Clin Psychiatry 2009;70(1):11–2.
73. Morrison MF, Kallan MJ, Ten Have T, et al. Lack of efficacy of estradiol for depression in postmenopausal women: a randomized, controlled trial. Biol Psychiatry 2004;55(4):406–12.
74. Morrison JH, Brinton RD, Schmidt PJ, et al. Estrogen, menopause, and the aging brain: how basic neuroscience can inform hormone therapy in women. J Neurosci 2006;26(41):10332–48.
75. Rudolph I, Palombo-Kinne E, Kirsch B, et al. Influence of a continuous combined HRT (2 mg estradiol valerate and 2 mg dienogest) on postmenopausal depression. Climacteric 2004;7(3):301–11.
76. Santoro N. The menopausal transition. Am J Med 2005;118(Suppl 12B):8–13.
77. Maki PM, Freeman EW, Greendale GA, et al. Summary of the National Institute on Aging-sponsored conference on depressive symptoms and cognitive complaints in the menopausal transition. Menopause 2010;17(4):815–22.
78. Freeman MP, Cheng LJ, Moustafa D, et al. Vortioxetine for major depressive disorder, vasomotor, and cognitive symptoms associated with the menopausal transition. Ann Clin Psychiatry 2017;29(4):249–57.
79. Frey BN, Haber E, Mendes GC, et al. Effects of quetiapine extended release on sleep and quality of life in midlife women with major depressive disorder. Arch Womens Ment Health 2013;16(1):83–5.
80. Gambacciani M, Ciaponi M, Cappagli B, et al. Effects of low-dose, continuous combined estradiol and noretisterone acetate on menopausal quality of life in early postmenopausal women. Maturitas 2003;44(2):157–63.
81. Joffe H, Groninger H, Soares CN, et al. An open trial of mirtazapine in menopausal women with depression unresponsive to estrogen replacement therapy. J Womens Health Gend Based Med 2001;10(10):999–1004.

82. Joffe H, Soares CN, Petrillo LF, et al. Treatment of depression and menopause-related symptoms with the serotonin-norepinephrine reuptake inhibitor duloxetine. J Clin Psychiatry 2007;68(6):943–50.
83. Kornstein SG, Jiang Q, Reddy S, et al. Short-term efficacy and safety of desvenlafaxine in a randomized, placebo-controlled study of perimenopausal and postmenopausal women with major depressive disorder. J Clin Psychiatry 2010;71(8):1088–96.
84. Soares CN, Kornstein SG, Thase ME, et al. Assessing the efficacy of desvenlafaxine for improving functioning and well-being outcome measures in patients with major depressive disorder: a pooled analysis of 9 double-blind, placebo-controlled, 8-week clinical trials. J Clin Psychiatry 2009;70(10):1365–71.
85. Soares CN, Thase ME, Clayton A, et al. Desvenlafaxine and escitalopram for the treatment of postmenopausal women with major depressive disorder. Menopause 2010;17(4):700–11.
86. Soares CN, Frey BN, Haber E, et al. A pilot, 8-week, placebo lead-in trial of quetiapine extended release for depression in midlife women: impact on mood and menopause-related symptoms. J Clin Psychopharmacol 2010;30(5):612–5.
87. Maki PM, Kornstein SG, Joffe H, et al, Board of Trustees for The North American Menopause Society (NAMS) and the Women and Mood Disorders Task Force of the National Network of Depression Centers. Guidelines for the evaluation and treatment of perimenopausal depression: summary and recommendations. Menopause 2018;25(10):1069–85.
88. Green SM, Key BL, McCabe RE. Cognitive-behavioral, behavioral, and mindfulness-based therapies for menopausal depression: a review. Maturitas 2015;80(1):37–47.

Update on Binge Eating Disorder

Anna I. Guerdjikova, PhD, LISW[a,b,*], Nicole Mori, RN, MSN, APRN-BC[a,b], Leah S. Casuto, MD[a,b], Susan L. McElroy, MD[a,b]

KEYWORDS

- Binge eating disorder • Female binge eating • Treatment • Gender • Sex differences
- Eating dysregulation

KEY POINTS

- Binge eating disorder is more prevalent than anorexia nervosa and bulimia nervosa combined and it is the most common eating disorder in males.
- Binge eating disorder remains underrecognized and undertreated in both sexes.
- Males and females with binge eating disorder are more similar than different in their presentation and treatment response.
- Binge eating disorder is a treatable illness and psychological and pharmacologic treatments are now available.

BINGE EATING DISORDER

Binge eating disorder (BED) is the most common eating disorder (ED) and an important public health problem worldwide. Recent data from the World Health Organization Mental Survey Study, which surveyed adults from 14 countries on 4 continents, found a lifetime prevalence rate of BED to be 1.4%.[1] Of note, BED is the most common ED is

This is an update of an article that first appeared in the *Psychiatric Clinics of North America*, Volume 40, Issue 2, June 2017.
N. Mori and L.S. Casuto have nothing to disclose. A.I. Guerdjikova is a consultant for Bracket and Avanir. S.L. McElroy has been a consultant to or member of the scientific advisory boards of Allergan, Avanir, Bracket, F. Hoffmann-La Roche Ltd., Mitsubishi Tanabe Pharma America, Myriad, Opiant, Shire, and Sunovion. She has been a principal or co-investigator on studies sponsored by Allergan, Avanir, Azevan, Brainsway, Marriott Foundation, Medibio, Myriad, Neurocrine, Novo Nordisk, Shire, and Sunovion. She is also an inventor on United States Patent No. 6,323,236 B2, Use of Sulfamate Derivatives for Treating Impulse Control Disorders, and along with the patent's assignee, University of Cincinnati, Cincinnati, Ohio, and has received payments from Johnson & Johnson, which has exclusive rights under the patent.
[a] Lindner Center of HOPE, 4075 Old Western Row Road, Mason, OH 45040, USA; [b] Department of Psychiatry and Behavioral Neuroscience, University of Cincinnati College of Medicine, 4075 Old Western Row Road, Mason, OH 45040, USA
* Corresponding author. Department of Psychiatry and Behavioral Neuroscience, Lindner Center of HOPE, University of Cincinnati College of Medicine, 4075 Old Western Row Road, Mason, OH 45040.
E-mail address: anna.guerdjikova@lindnercenter.org

Med Clin N Am 103 (2019) 669–680
http://dx.doi.org/10.1016/j.mcna.2019.02.003 medical.theclinics.com
0025-7125/19/

adolescence. It is estimated to occur in up to 1.3% of adolescents in the US general population[2] and its prevalence tends to increase overtime in both males and females.[3] BED continues to be an underrecognized and undertreated condition. Patients rarely spontaneously disclose binge-eating symptoms because of embarrassment or shame. Binge-eating behavior is overlooked, and treatment commonly focuses on obesity and its complications as the presenting problem rather than addressing the core eating psychopathology.

BED is characterized by recurrent episodes of binge eating, defined as eating in a discrete period of time (about 2 hours) an amount of food larger than most people would eat under similar circumstances and having a sense of loss of control over the eating. Additionally, patients do not engage in the inappropriate compensatory behaviors of bulimia nervosa (BN), for example, self-induced vomiting or excessive use of diuretic or laxatives. Binge-eating episodes are associated with feelings of guilt and distress and occur on average at least once a week for 3 consecutive months. During a binge-eating episode, patients might eat large amounts of food when not feeling physically hungry, eat more rapidly than normal, and eat until feeling uncomfortably full. Patients with BED often eat in secrecy; they are embarrassed by the binge-eating behavior and their perceived inability to control the urges to overeat.[4]

HISTORICAL OVERVIEW OF BINGE EATING DISORDER AND OTHER EATING DISORDERS

Anorexia nervosa (AN), BN, and BED are the 3 major types of EDs outlined in *Diagnostic and Statistical Manual of Mental Disorders*, fifth edition (*DSM-5*).[4] AN is characterized by intense fear of gaining weight or becoming fat resulting in persistent restriction of food intake leading to significantly low body weight. Individuals with BN engage in recurrent binge-eating behaviors followed by inappropriate compensatory weight-loss behaviors, such as self-induced vomiting or abuse of laxatives or diuretics. BED is characterized by recurrent episodes of binge eating that are not followed by the inappropriate weight loss behaviors diagnostic for BN. The estimated lifetime prevalence of *DSM-IV* AN, BN, and BED is 0.9%, 1.5%, and 3.5% among women and 0.3% 0.5%, and 2.0% among men, respectively[5]; thus, BED is more common than AN and BN combined. All EDs are highly heritable illnesses[6] and associated with decreased quality of life and increased disability, morbidity, and mortality.[1,7]

Medical cases describing symptoms of AN appeared in literature in the early seventeenth century with the work of the English physician Dr Morton. Binging with subsequent purging were both known through ancient history with the Hebrew Talmud (AD 400–500) referring to a ravenous hunger that should be treated with sweet foods (boolmot), but the medical term *bulimia nervosa* was not introduced until 1979 and then included as a formal diagnosis in *DSM-III* in 1987. BED was first formally described in 1959 by Albert Stunkard[8] as a form of abnormal eating among obese patients. In his seminal article "Eating Patterns and Obesity," he described a female patient with binge eating as follows: "She usually began to feel a desire for food in the early evening, and would eat a large supper. Only temporarily sated, she soon returned to the kitchen and consumed larger and larger amounts of food at progressively shorter intervals. During these hours, she was assailed by loneliness and anxiety. She rarely fell asleep before midnight, and usually awoke within an hour, anxious and hungry. Then she would eat a pint of ice cream and drink a bottle of soda pop."[8]

Overall, all 3 types of EDs received little systematic attention until the middle of the twentieth century when they were conceptualized as mental illnesses and included in formal disease classifications. As recently as 2013, BED was added to *DSM-5* as a stand-alone psychiatric disorder.

OVERVIEW OF PSYCHIATRIC AND MEDICAL COMORBIDITIES OF BINGE EATING DISORDER

BED co-occurs with a plethora of psychiatric disorders, most commonly mood and anxiety disorders. Data from 9282 participants in the National Comorbidity Survey demonstrated that approximately 4 out of 5 adults with lifetime BED have at least one comorbid psychiatric disorder, and approximately 1 out of 2 adults with BED has 3 or more comorbid psychiatric disorders.[5] Consistently, in a study of 404 patients with BED, 73.8% had at least one additional lifetime psychiatric disorder and 43.1% had at least one current psychiatric disorder.[9] Mood (54.2%), anxiety (37.1%), and substance use (24.8%) disorders were the most common psychiatric disorders among patients with BED. Of interest, in a recent study among 11,588 adult men and women presenting to ED treatment clinics in Sweden, the highest levels of psychiatric comorbidity were among women with BED as compared with women with AN and BN, particularly regarding anxiety (55%) and mood (45%) disorders.[10]

Obesity and its complications are among the medical comorbidities most commonly associated with BED. Growing evidence suggests that BED may independently increase the risk of development of certain components of metabolic syndrome, like diabetes, hypertension, and dyslipidemia, over and above the risk attributable to obesity alone.[11] Other medical disorders or problems with BED include pain condition, sleep disorders and sleep problems, fibromyalgia, and irritable bowel syndrome.[12] Preliminary data indicate that the cardiovascular system, reproductive system, and cortisol response might also be affected in patients with BED.[13]

BINGE EATING DISORDER IN WOMEN VERSUS BINGE EATING DISORDER IN MEN

In contrast to AN and BN, which occur in a 9:1 female to male ratio, the female to male ratio is more balanced in BED, about 6:4.[5] Sex disparities in EDs have been hypothesized to be due to the interplay between biological differences between women and men and to the differential influence of sociocultural factors on the sexes. Among biological differences, the organizational effect of estrogens during puberty is thought to facilitate the development of BEDs in genetically vulnerable females.[14] Binge eating frequency and dysfunctional eating symptoms are higher during the luteal phase of the menstrual cycle; correlations between estradiol and progesterone levels and disordered eating were demonstrated across levels of dietary restraint, levels of impulsivity, and patients' body mass index (BMI).[15] From a sociocultural perspective, overvaluation of the "thin ideal" and increased exposure to dieting and peer pressure might preferentially increase the risk for EDs in females.[16]

Five studies have compared the features of males and females with BED in clinical samples.[17–21] Interestingly, males and females with BED consistently seem to be more similar than different in their presentations. In the first study, baseline characteristics of 21 men and 21 age-matched women with BED were compared using the Eating Disorders Examination (EDE), the Structured Clinical Interview for *DSM-III-R* (SCID), and SCID II for personality disorder assessments.[17] Men and women did not differ on measures of eating disturbance, shape and weight concerns, interpersonal problems, or self-esteem. Although women were more likely to report eating in response to negative emotions, particularly anger, frustration, and anxiety, more men met criteria for at least one axis I diagnosis and had a lifetime diagnosis of substance dependence. In the second study, 35 men and 147 women who were consecutively evaluated for outpatient clinical trials in BED were administered a battery of measures to examine developmental, eating and weight-related disturbances, and psychological features associated with BED.[19] Men and women did not differ significantly on developmental variables or on measures of current ED features, like binge-eating behaviors or weight or shape concerns. However, higher body dissatisfaction, drive for thinness, dietary restraint, and emotional eating were significantly more prevalent among women. In the third study, 44 obese men with BED were compared with 44 age- and race-matched obese women with BED seeking weight-loss treatment.[18] Obese men with BED had attempted significantly fewer diets and used fewer medications and supplements for weight loss, but the two sexes did not differ significantly in ages of onset of BED or obesity, current BMI, number of binge-eating episodes at presentation for treatment, or presence or severity of mood disorder symptoms. In the fourth study, 198 obese adults (26% men) were recruited in primary care settings for a treatment study for obesity and BED.[20] Women reported significantly earlier age at onset of overweight and dieting and greater frequency of dieting, and men engaged in more frequent strenuous exercise. Men were also more likely than women to meet criteria for metabolic syndrome. However, women and men did not differ on onset for either overweight or binge eating or in features of EDs, emotional eating scores, perceived stress, depressive symptoms, or self-control. In the fifth study, data were pooled from 408 women and 54 men who were participants in pharmacotherapy trials for BED.[21] Men and women with BED who enrolled in pharmacotherapy studies were similar on most variables, including age of onset of BED and severity of BED symptoms. However, men were older at study entry, had lower levels of depressive symptoms, and had a greater frequency of lifetime alcohol use disorders. Additionally, men had significantly higher BMIs, significantly higher systolic and diastolic blood pressures, and were taking more prescription medications for diabetes and dyslipidemia.

The few studies that have examined sex differences in BED treatment outcome have not found significant differences.[18,21–24] Of interest, a recent study aggregated data from 11 randomized controlled psychosocial BED treatment studies and examined differences between 208 men and 1117 women. Baseline and outcome symptoms were assessed via the interview and questionnaire versions of the EDE. Men and women reported similar levels of dietary restraint and binge-eating episode frequencies at baseline. Men reported significantly lower shape, weight, and eating concerns as well as lower global EDE scores than women. After treatment, men and women did not differ significantly on global EDE score, number of binge-eating episodes in the past 28 days, remission of binge eating, or premature study dropout.[25] Similarly, in the review of 9 double-blind, placebo-controlled, randomized trials and 2 open-label trials examining various medications for BED, of 88 participants receiving an antidepressant, 66% of the women and 88% the men were responders. Of the 80 participants receiving an antiepileptic medication, 74% of women and 80% of men were responders with no significant differences between the two sexes.[21] In sum, limited available data suggest women and men with BED are more similar than different in their presentation and response to psychological and pharmacologic treatments.

NEUROBIOLOGY OF BINGE EATING DISORDER IN WOMEN

Sex differences in eating behavior have been the subject of physiologic research over the last century since the initial observations that the removal of the ovaries leads to accumulation of adipose tissue and that food intake varies through the ovarian cycle in intact female rats. Appetite and satiety variations across the menstrual cycle have been documented in women.[26,27] Additionally, there are sex differences in sensory and flavor hedonic responses.[28,29] These differences in eating are thought to be mediated by a complex network including cholecystokinin, glucagonlike peptide-1, glucagon, insulin, amylin, apolipoprotein, and leptin orchestrated by the central neurochemical signaling via serotonin and glutamate and numerous neuropeptides.[15]

Study of the neurobiology of BED in humans is in its infancy. For example, females with BED have shown greater cognitive attentional biases toward food; decreased reward sensitivities; cognitive deficits in attention, executive function inhibitory control, and decision making; and altered brain activation in regions associated with impulsivity and.[30] Right-insular cortex activation differentiates women with BED from obese and normal-weight non-BED women.[31] Neurophysiologic and neuroimaging studies comparing obese women with BED with non-BED obese women suggested that altered function in cortical and striatal brain regions possibly contributes to BED. For example, increased centroparietal cortical long-latency event-related potentials when viewing high-caloric food[32] and increased regional cerebral blood flow in left frontal and prefrontal cortices in response to food stimuli[33] have been observed in obese females with BED compared with similarly obese females without BED.

Although most studies of BED neurobiology have been done in females, the effects of ovarian hormones on eating behavior and weight regulation have not been empirically determined. Ovarian hormones might exhibit a genomic effect within the central nervous system as they act as gene transcription factors in several neurobiological systems that are known to be related to deregulated eating behavior.[34] High levels of progesterone and low levels of estradiol were reported to be associated with increased binge eating and emotional eating in a nonclinical sample of 19 healthy women[35] and in women with BN.[36] Furthermore, estradiol and progesterone interaction might predict within-person changes in emotional eating, independent of negative effect and BMI.[37] Work by the same group also demonstrated that low estradiol and low progesterone were associated with greater dysregulated eating in women with objective binge-eating episodes, in addition to the high estradiol and high progesterone risk milieu.[38]

MEDICAL COMORBIDITY OF BINGE EATING DISORDER IN WOMEN

It is well established that BED is associated with obesity.[5] Moreover, binge-eating behavior is prospectively associated with the development of obesity.[39,40]

The authors were able to locate 6 cross-sectional studies of various medical conditions in women with BED, and they are summarized in **Table 1**. Among women, BED is associated with early menarche, menstrual dysfunction, delivery of higher-birth-weight babies, and long duration of the first and second stages of labor.[41–44]

Conversely, certain endocrine conditions in women might be associated with BED. Among 215 women with type 2 diabetes, 13.5% had *DSM-IV* BED and binge eating predicted blood glucose control after controlling for BMI and exercise level.[45] In another study, women with type 2 diabetes and BED had a significantly higher BMI and A1C levels than diabetic controls without BED.[46] Among 103 women with polycystic ovary syndrome, 13% had BED compared with 2% of controls.[47] Finally, metabolic syndrome has been reported to be more common in men with BED than women with BED[48,49]; but this finding is inconsistent.[18,50]

TREATMENT OF BINGE EATING DISORDER IN WOMEN

BED remains underrecognized and undertreated. Primary care doctors are often unaware of the disorder. A decade old survey of physicians reported that more than 40% had never assessed their patients for BED.[51] Only one-third of patients with BED and BN had been asked about problems with eating by their primary care or other health care professional,[52] and less than 10% of respondents with BED received treatment of their ED within the last year.[1]

Table 1
Cross-sectional studies of medical conditions in women with binge eating disorder

Study	Participants	Assessments	Findings
Johnson et al,[44] 2001	4651 Female patients	Patient Health Questionnaire and General Health Survey	Women with BED were significantly more likely to have diabetes. BED was also associated with increased prevalence of menstrual problems, shortness of breath, chest pain, limb or joint pain, headaches, and gastrointestinal problems,
Bulik et al,[62] 2002	166 Caucasian obese female twins	Symptom checklist	BE was not associated with hypertension, visual impairment, asthma/respiratory illness, DM, cardiac problems, osteoarthritis, or any major medical disorder as compared with no BE.
Trace et al,[63] 2012	Population-base sample of 3790 female Swedish twins	Questionnaire about sleep habits	Lifetime BE was significantly associated with not getting enough sleep. The associations between BE and sleep remained after accounting for obesity.
Algars et al,[41] 2014	11,503 Swedish female twins	Evaluation for menstrual dysfunctions	BE, but not BED, was significantly associated with lifetime oligomenorrhea and amenorrhea.
Linna et al,[42] 2014	2257 Female patients with ED	Registry on pregnancy, obstetric, and perinatal health	Women with BED had babies with higher birth weight, and maternal BED was associated with hypertension.
Rosenbaum et al,[64] 2016	484 Female primary care patients	Patient Health Questionnaire and review of medical history	Women with BED had significantly higher rates of chronic pain, lipid disorders, hypertension, and sleep disorders.

Abbreviations: BE, binge eating behavior; DM, diabetes.

A variety of clinician-administered or self-report tools to aid diagnosing of BED have been recently developed. For example, a validated self-report screening instrument for BED has been developed by Shire Inc (Binge Eating Disorder Screener-7) and is available free of charge on their BED educational portal. Other instruments that can be used for BED screening and diagnosis include Binge Eating Scale[53] and the Eating Disorder Examination-Questionnaire.[54] Several government institutions and not-for-profit organizations offer support to patients with BED and provide resources for health care professionals. A comprehensive list of resources for professionals and patients is listed in **Table 2**.

Psychotherapy alone or in combination with self-help tools can be considered the first line of treatment, especially if BED signs and symptoms are mild and there are no clinically significant psychiatric comorbidities.[55] It is recommended that all patients seeking treatment of BED should receive psychoeducation.[56] Cognitive behavior psychotherapy (CBT), interpersonal therapy, and to a lesser degree dialectical behavior therapy are the specific psychotherapies that have been effective for reducing binge-eating symptoms and associated psychopathology. Their psychotherapies are not effective, however, for weight loss in these patients.[57] A basic feature of CBT is developing awareness of one's eating behaviors by daily monitoring and recording of problematic behaviors. Numerous applications for mobile devices have been developed in the recent years as self-help tools or to enhance treatment of EDs.[58]

In moderate and severe BED cases, pharmacotherapy can be considered as monotherapy or in conjunction with psychological interventions. Various classes of medications, including antidepressants, antiepileptic drugs, antiobesity drugs, and medications approved for attention-deficit/hyperactivity disorder (ADHD), have been tested in randomized placebo-controlled trials in BED and found helpful in improving binge-eating behavior and eating-related psychopathology.[57] The only medication that has regulatory approval for treatment of BED is lisdexamfetamine dimesylate (LDX). LDX is specifically approved for treatment of adults with moderate to severe BED. This approval was based on 3 randomized placebo-controlled studies in acute adult BED: an 11-week phase II proof-of-concept study and 2 identically designed 12-week phase III trials enrolling a total of 1044 patients. LDX dosed at 50 mg or 70 mg (but not 30 mg) significantly reduced binge-eating symptoms, obsessive-compulsive features of binge eating, and other measures of EDs psychopathology. Adverse reactions reported by 3% or more of adult patients with ADHD taking LDX and at least twice the incidence compared with patients taking placebo included decreased appetite, insomnia, dry mouth, diarrhea, nausea, anxiety, anorexia, feeling jittery, agitation, increased blood pressure, hyperhidrosis, restlessness and decrease weight. In the United States, the Drug Enforcement Administration categorizes LDX as a schedule II medication; thus, risk of abuse and dependence requires close monitoring. Moreover, although LDX was associated with weight loss in the 3 clinical trials, it is not approved for weight loss or treatment of obesity.

As already reviewed, BED is often comorbid with other psychiatric conditions. Females, in particular, often present for treatment with nonspecific mixed symptoms of chronic low mood, general anxiety, consistent weight gain or a pattern of yo-yo dieting, sleep disturbances, poor concentration, and anhedonia. Carefully diagnosing potential mood disorders and treating them accordingly is of paramount importance in the management of BED. Women with a mood disorder and a co-occurring BED commonly present with multidimensional problems that often cannot be treated with a single intervention and benefit from a team approach to management to optimize outcomes. Ideally, a team of professionals, including a psychiatrist, a dietician, and a therapist, would be available to provide support for patients and their families.

Table 2
Resources for professionals and patients

Resource	Web Site/Portal	Resource Helpful for
Academy for Eating Disorders (AED)	http://www.aedweb.org/	Clinicians
National Institute of Diabetes and Digestive and Kidney Diseases (NIDDK)	https://www.niddk.nih.gov/health-information/	Clinicians
International Journal for Eating Disorders	http://onlinelibrary.wiley.com/journal/10.1002/(ISSN)1098-108X	Clinicians
National Eating Disorders Collaboration	http://nedc.com.au/about-the-nedc	Clinicians and patients
WebMD	http://www.webmd.com/	Clinicians and patients
Understanding Binge Eating	http://www.bingeeatingdisorder.com/	Clinicians and patients
Binge Eating Disorder Association (BEDA)	http://bedaonline.com/	Clinicians and patients
National Eating Disorder Association (NEDA)	http://www.nationaleatingdisorders.org/	Clinicians and patients
Mobile Device Apps[a]	Recovery Record (iPhone) Rise Up (Android)	Clinicians and patients

Abbreviation: apps, applications.
[a] The two applications (apps) listed are the most downloaded and widely used.[58] There are more than 50 apps available with an ED focus and 10 or more specifically designed for BED. For a comprehensive list, please refer to "Apps and eating disorders: A systematic clinical appraisal."[58]

In regard to medical comorbidity, patients diagnosed with BED should receive comprehensive medical evaluations with particular focus on diabetes, hypertension, dyslipidemias, pain, sleep disorders, functional gastrointestinal disorders, and asthma; women should additionally receive evaluation of reproductive function and for polycystic ovary syndrome.

Finally, bariatric surgery has been shown to be effective for the treatment of severe obesity; a notable proportion of bariatric surgery candidates had loss-of-control eating or BED.[59] Among bariatric surgery candidates, there were no differences in BED rates or binge eating between women and men[60] and weight loss and metabolic outcomes after bariatric surgery were of similar magnitude in both sexes.[61]

SUMMARY

In summary, BED is the most prevalent ED but it continues to be underrecognized and undertreated. BED is more common in females than in males but to a lesser degree than AN and BN. Presentation and response to treatment of BED in females and males is more similar than dissimilar, but this area requires further study. Neurochemical correlates of EDs in general, and of BED in particular, are a growing field of basic and clinical research that will help elucidate the biological substrate in those disorders and further guide treatment. Recent validation of BED as a stand-alone diagnosis in *DSM-5* and approval of the first medication for its treatment mark the beginning of a new era in the comprehensive management of BED.

REFERENCES

1. Kessler RC, Berglund PA, Chiu WT, et al. The prevalence and correlates of binge eating disorder in the World Health Organization World Mental Health Surveys. Biol Psychiatry 2013;73(9):904–14.
2. Swanson SA, Crow SJ, Le Grange D, et al. Prevalence and correlates of eating disorders in adolescents. Results from the national comorbidity survey replication adolescent supplement. Arch Gen Psychiatry 2011;68(7):714–23.
3. Marzilli E, Cerniglia L, Cimino S. A narrative review of binge eating disorder in adolescence: prevalence, impact, and psychological treatment strategies. Adolesc Health Med Ther 2018;9:17–30.
4. American Psychiatric Association. Diagnostic and statistical manual of mental disorders. 5th edition. Arlington (VA): American Psychiatric Publishing; 2013. p. 2013.
5. Hudson JI, Hiripi E, Pope HG Jr, et al. The prevalence and correlates of eating disorders in the National Comorbidity Survey Replication. Biol Psychiatry 2007; 61(3):348–58.
6. Tozzi F, Bulik CM. Candidate genes in eating disorders. Curr Drug Targets CNS Neurol Disord 2003;2(1):31–9.
7. Fichter MM, Quadflieg N. Mortality in eating disorders - results of a large prospective clinical longitudinal study. Int J Eat Disord 2016;49(4):391–401.
8. Stunkard AJ. Eating patterns and obesity. Psychiatr Q 1959;33:284–95.
9. Grilo CM, White MA, Masheb RM. DSM-IV psychiatric disorder comorbidity and its correlates in binge eating disorder. Int J Eat Disord 2009;42(3):228–34.
10. Ulfvebrand S, Birgegard A, Norring C, et al. Psychiatric comorbidity in women and men with eating disorders results from a large clinical database. Psychiatry Res 2015;230(2):294–9.
11. Hudson JI, Lalonde JK, Coit CE, et al. Longitudinal study of the diagnosis of components of the metabolic syndrome in individuals with binge-eating disorder. Am J Clin Nutr 2010;91(6):1568–73.

12. Olguin P, Fuentes M, Gabler G, et al. Medical comorbidity of binge eating disorder. Eat Weight Disord 2016. [Epub ahead of print].
13. Mitchell JE. Medical comorbidity and medical complications associated with binge-eating disorder. Int J Eat Disord 2016;49(3):319–23.
14. Culbert KM, Racine SE, Klump KL. The influence of gender and puberty on the heritability of disordered eating symptoms. Curr Top Behav Neurosci 2011;6:177–85.
15. Asarian L, Geary N. Sex differences in the physiology of eating. Am J Physiol Regul Integr Comp Physiol 2013;305(11):R1215–67.
16. Urquhart CS, Mihalynuk TV. Disordered eating in women: implications for the obesity pandemic. Can J Diet Pract Res 2011;72(1):e115–25.
17. Tanofsky MB, Wilfley DE, Spurrell EB, et al. Comparison of men and women with binge eating disorder. Int J Eat Disord 1997;21(1):49–54.
18. Guerdjikova AI, McElroy SL, Kotwal R, et al. Comparison of obese men and women with binge eating disorder seeking weight management. Eat Weight Disord 2007;12(1):e19–23.
19. Barry DT, Grilo CM, Masheb RM. Gender differences in patients with binge eating disorder. Int J Eat Disord 2002;31(1):63–70.
20. Udo T, McKee SA, White MA, et al. Sex differences in biopsychosocial correlates of binge eating disorder: a study of treatment-seeking obese adults in primary care setting. Gen Hosp Psychiatry 2013;35(6):587–91.
21. Guerdjikova A, Blom TJ, Mori N, et al. Gender differences in binge eating disorder: a pooled analysis of eleven pharmacotherapy trials from one research group. J Mens Health 2014;11(4):183–8.
22. Munsch S, Biedert E, Meyer A, et al. A randomized comparison of cognitive behavioral therapy and behavioral weight loss treatment for overweight individuals with binge eating disorder. Int J Eat Disord 2007;40(2):102–13.
23. Safer DL, Robinson AH, Jo B. Outcome from a randomized controlled trial of group therapy for binge eating disorder: comparing dialectical behavior therapy adapted for binge eating to an active comparison group therapy. Behav Ther 2010;41(1):106–20.
24. Ricca V, Castellini G, Mannucci E, et al. Comparison of individual and group cognitive behavioral therapy for binge eating disorder. A randomized, three-year follow-up study. Appetite 2010;55(3):656–65.
25. Shingleton RM, Thompson-Brenner H, Thompson DR, et al. Gender differences in clinical trials of binge eating disorder: an analysis of aggregated data. J Consult Clin Psychol 2015;83(2):382–6.
26. Pohle-Krauza RJ, Carey KH, Pelkman CL. Dietary restraint and menstrual cycle phase modulated L-phenylalanine-induced satiety. Physiol Behav 2008;93(4–5):851–61.
27. Geiker NR, Ritz C, Pedersen SD, et al. A weight-loss program adapted to the menstrual cycle increases weight loss in healthy, overweight, premenopausal women: a 6-mo randomized controlled trial. Am J Clin Nutr 2016;104(1):15–20.
28. Hayes JE, Duffy VB. Oral sensory phenotype identifies level of sugar and fat required for maximal liking. Physiol Behav 2008;95(1–2):77–87.
29. Drewnowski A, Kurth C, Holden-Wiltse J, et al. Food preferences in human obesity: carbohydrates versus fats. Appetite 1992;18(3):207–21.
30. Kessler RM, Hutson PH, Herman BK, et al. The neurobiological basis of binge-eating disorder. Neurosci Biobehav Rev 2016;63:223–38.
31. Weygandt M, Schaefer A, Schienle A, et al. Diagnosing different binge-eating disorders based on reward-related brain activation patterns. Hum Brain Mapp 2012;33(9):2135–46.

32. Svaldi J, Tuschen-Caffier B, Peyk P, et al. Information processing of food pictures in binge eating disorder. Appetite 2010;55(3):685–94.
33. Karhunen LJ, Vanninen EJ, Kuikka JT, et al. Regional cerebral blood flow during exposure to food in obese binge eating women. Psychiatry Res 2000;99(1):29–42.
34. Ostlund H, Keller E, Hurd YL. Estrogen receptor gene expression in relation to neuropsychiatric disorders. Ann N Y Acad Sci 2003;1007:54–63.
35. Klump KL, Keel PK, Culbert KM, et al. Ovarian hormones and binge eating: exploring associations in community samples. Psychol Med 2008;38(12):1749–57.
36. Edler C, Lipson SF, Keel PK. Ovarian hormones and binge eating in bulimia nervosa. Psychol Med 2007;37(1):131–41.
37. Klump KL, Keel PK, Racine SE, et al. The interactive effects of estrogen and progesterone on changes in emotional eating across the menstrual cycle. J Abnorm Psychol 2013;122(1):131–7.
38. Klump KL, Racine SE, Hildebrandt B, et al. Ovarian hormone influences on dysregulated eating: a comparison of associations in women with versus without binge episodes. Clin Psychol Sci 2014;2(4):545–59.
39. Sonneville KR, Horton NJ, Micali N, et al. Longitudinal associations between binge eating and overeating and adverse outcomes among adolescents and young adults: does loss of control matter? JAMA Pediatr 2013;167(2):149–55.
40. Field AE, Sonneville KR, Micali N, et al. Prospective association of common eating disorders and adverse outcomes. Pediatrics 2012;130(2):e289–95.
41. Algars M, Huang L, Von Holle AF, et al. Binge eating and menstrual dysfunction. J Psychosom Res 2014;76(1):19–22.
42. Linna MS, Raevuori A, Haukka J, et al. Pregnancy, obstetric, and perinatal health outcomes in eating disorders. Am J Obstet Gynecol 2014;211(4):392.e1-8.
43. Reichborn-Kjennerud T, Bulik CM, Sullivan PF, et al. Psychiatric and medical symptoms in binge eating in the absence of compensatory behaviors. Obes Res 2004;12(9):1445–54.
44. Johnson JG, Spitzer RL, Williams JB. Health problems, impairment and illnesses associated with bulimia nervosa and binge eating disorder among primary care and obstetric gynaecology patients. Psychol Med 2001;31(8):1455–66.
45. Kenardy J, Mensch M, Bowen K, et al. A comparison of eating behaviors in newly diagnosed NIDDM patients and case-matched control subjects. Diabetes Care 1994;17(10):1197–9.
46. Takii M, Komaki G, Uchigata Y, et al. Differences between bulimia nervosa and binge-eating disorder in females with type 1 diabetes: the important role of insulin omission. J Psychosom Res 1999;47(3):221–31.
47. Hollinrake E, Abreu A, Maifeld M, et al. Increased risk of depressive disorders in women with polycystic ovary syndrome. Fertil Steril 2007;87(6):1369–76.
48. Barnes RD, Boeka AG, McKenzie KC, et al. Metabolic syndrome in obese patients with binge-eating disorder in primary care clinics: a cross-sectional study. Prim Care Companion CNS Disord 2011;13(2):PCC.10m01050.
49. Udo T, McKee SA, White MA, et al. Menopause and metabolic syndrome in obese individuals with binge eating disorder. Eat Behav 2014;15(2):182–5.
50. Blomquist KK, Milsom VA, Barnes RD, et al. Metabolic syndrome in obese men and women with binge eating disorder: developmental trajectories of eating and weight-related behaviors. Compr Psychiatry 2012;53(7):1021–7.
51. Crow SJ, Peterson CB, Levine AS, et al. A survey of binge eating and obesity treatment practices among primary care providers. Int J Eat Disord 2004;35(3):348–53.

52. Mond JM, Myers TC, Crosby RD, et al. Bulimic eating disorders in primary care: hidden morbidity still? J Clin Psychol Med Settings. 2010;17(1):56–63.
53. Gormally J, Black S, Daston S, et al. The assessment of binge eating severity among obese persons. Addict Behav 1982;7(1):47–55.
54. Fairburn CG, Beglin SJ. Assessment of eating disorders: interview or self-report questionnaire? Int J Eat Disord 1994;16(4):363–70.
55. Vocks S, Tuschen-Caffier B, Pietrowsky R, et al. Meta-analysis of the effectiveness of psychological and pharmacological treatments for binge eating disorder. Int J Eat Disord 2010;43(3):205–17.
56. Berkman ND, Brownley KA, Peat CM, et al. Management and outcomes of binge-eating disorder. Rockville (MD): Agency for Healthcare Research and Quality; 2015.
57. McElroy SL, Guerdjikova AI, Mori N, et al. Overview of the treatment of binge eating disorder. CNS Spectr 2015;20(6):546–56.
58. Fairburn CG, Rothwell ER. Apps and eating disorders: a systematic clinical appraisal. Int J Eat Disord 2015;48(7):1038–46.
59. Mitchell JE, King WC, Courcoulas A, et al. Eating behavior and eating disorders in adults before bariatric surgery. Int J Eat Disord 2015;48(2):215–22.
60. Mazzeo SE, Saunders R, Mitchell KS. Gender and binge eating among bariatric surgery candidates. Eat Behav 2006;7(1):47–52.
61. Kennedy-Dalby A, Adam S, Ammori BJ, et al. Weight loss and metabolic outcomes of bariatric surgery in men versus women - a matched comparative observational cohort study. Eur J Intern Med 2014;25(10):922–5.
62. Bulik CM, Sullivan PF, Kendler KS. Medical and psychiatric morbidity in obese women with and without binge eating. Int J Eat Disord 2002;32(1):72–8.
63. Trace SE, Thornton LM, Runfola CD, et al. Sleep problems are associated with binge eating in women. Int J Eat Disord 2012;45(5):695–703.
64. Rosenbaum DL, Kimerling R, Pomernacki A, et al. Binge eating among women veterans in primary care: comorbidities and treatment priorities. Womens Health Issues 2016;26(4):420–8.

Female Sexual Dysfunction

Anita H. Clayton, MD*, Elia Margarita Valladares Juarez, MD

KEYWORDS

- Female sexual dysfunction • Hypoactive sexual desire disorder
- Sexual arousal disorder • Female sexual pain disorder

KEY POINTS

- Diagnostic categories for female sexual disorders are discussed as well as a review of the clinical utility and current categories, including the *International Classification of Diseases, Eleventh Revision*; the *Diagnostic and Statistical Manual of Mental Disorders* (Fifth Edition); the International Consultation on Sexual Medicine; and other nomenclature systems.
- Definitions of sexual dysfunctions in women and epidemiologic data of female sexual dysfunctions currently available are discussed.
- Evidence-based diagnosis and treatment supported by the literature, other clinical guidelines and principles and experts' consensus recommendations are reviewed.

The aim of this article is to discuss the different types, classifications, causes, and treatment modalities of female sexual dysfunction (FSD). The topics of discussion include

- Nosology of FSD
- Classification systems and nomenclature in the field, including the International Consultation in Sexual Medicine (ICSM), International Society for the Study of Vulvovaginal Disease (ISSVD), *Diagnostic and Statistical Manual of Mental Disorders* (Fourth Edition) (*DSM-IV*) and *Diagnostic and Statistical Manual of Mental Disorders* (Fifth Edition) (*DSM-5*), and *International Classification of Diseases, Tenth Revision* (*ICD-10*) and the proposed *International Classification of Diseases and Related Health Problems* (*ICD-11*)
- Overview of FSD, differential diagnosis, and management

This article originally appeared in the *Psychiatric Clinics of North America*, Volume 40, Issue 2, June 2017.
E.M. Valladares Juarez has nothing to disclose. A.H. Clayton: Grants: Endoceutics, Inc.; Janssen; Sage Therapeutics; Takeda. Advisory Board Fee/Consultant Fee: Acadia; Alkermes; Allergan; AMAG Pharmaceuticals, Inc.; Fabre-Kramer; Lundbeck; Otsuka; Palatin Technologies; S1 Biopharma; Sage Therapeutics; Sprout Pharmaceuticals; Takeda. Royalties/Copyright: Ballantine Books/Random House; Changes in Sexual Functioning Questionnaire; Guilford Publications. Shares/Restricted Stock Units: Euthymics; S1 Biopharma.
Department of Psychiatry and Neurobehavioral Sciences, University of Virginia Health System, P.O. Box 800623, Charlottesville, VA 22908-0623, USA
* Corresponding author.
E-mail address: AHC8V@hscmail.mcc.virginia.edu

Med Clin N Am 103 (2019) 681–698
http://dx.doi.org/10.1016/j.mcna.2019.02.008
medical.theclinics.com

CHANGES IN DIAGNOSTIC CATEGORIES

In 2013, changes to diagnostic categories were proposed for FSDs in the new version of the *DSM-5*. The changes include

- The previous categories of female hypoactive sexual desire disorder (HSDD) and female sexual arousal disorder (FSAD) were combined into a new category called female sexual interest/arousal disorder (FSIAD).
- The separate diagnoses of dyspareunia and vaginismus were merged into a single diagnosis of genito-pelvic pain/penetration disorder (GPPD).
- Sexual aversion disorder, a diagnosis thought by the *DSM-5* committee to have limited empirical support and with more similarities to anxiety disorders and phobias, was eliminated.[1]
- Frequency and severity criteria were included in diagnostic criteria with potential to enhance clinical research.[2]
- Diagnoses are sex specific.

Overall the changes in *DSM-5* represent a departure from nosology based on presumed cause to a condensation of diagnoses based on groups of conditions with common symptoms or syndromes. Unfortunately, comorbidity of diagnoses does not mean the diagnoses are the same (eg, major depressive disorder and anxiety disorders have 50% comorbidity but are not merged in *DSM-5*).

All of these new classifications have duration and severity criteria with the exception of substance/medication-induced sexual dysfunction. The subtypes of lifelong versus acquired, generalized versus situational, and due to psychological factors versus combined factors have also been changed. Sexual dysfunction due to a general medical condition and the subtype due to psychological versus combined factors were eliminated.

It is unclear whether these changes represent a simplification from the previous *DSM-IV-TR* (Text Revision) version or if they accurately represent a common etiologic root for these disorders. Proponents of the new criteria have pointed out that *DSM-IV-TR* was based on a linear model of the human sexual response cycle based on the work of Masters and Johnson[3] dating from 1966 and that the human sexual response is not always linear (~5%–25% of men and women report a nonlinear model of sexual function as representative of their sexual response).[4–6] The phases of the sexual response cycle previously used may, therefore, be artificial for some individuals (eg, desire vs arousal).

Both *DSM-IV-TR* and *DSM-5* classification systems have limitations. There is a high level of false negatives. Both systems fail to identify most individuals who report sexual difficulties.[7] Use of a check-box template and lumping of diagnoses as in *DSM-V* reduces diagnostic specificity/precision.[8] Additionally, there are no data to support physiologic differences in sexual function between the sexes (except for physical/genital manifestations of arousal). Because of these limitations, experts in sexual medicine have proposed a revision of the current criteria, arguing that improved definitions and criteria encompassing all models of sexual response and across both sexes would better address issues related to accurate identification of individuals with sexual dysfunction and be useful to investigators for research purposes.

Challenges in identification and treatment of FSD include women's discomfort with the topic, reproductive-focused cultures, inadequate clinician training, and limited available time to elicit an in-depth sexual history. Clinicians must be able to differentiate between sexual disorders and transient states secondary to situational factors, such as relationship conflict and other temporary sexual problems that may represent variants of normal sexual functioning. Therefore, a clear and precise definition remains critical for the diagnosis and treatment of these conditions and to avoid medicalization of normal human sexual response and experience.[9]

The *DSM-5* criteria for sexual dysfunction require a minimum duration of 6 months of symptoms. Those symptoms must be present 75% to 100% of the time for all diagnoses, with the exception of medication- and substance-induced sexual dysfunction. This criterion eliminates inclusion of individuals with mild to moderate symptoms and renders the severity rating specifier pointless. Also, symptoms must cause significant distress in the individual.

Table 1 represents a comparison of the changes that took place between the *DSM-IV-TR*[10] and *DSM-5*[11] categories.

The *ICD-11* is under development with the goal to enhance clinical utility, provide clearly organized and consistent information across disorders, and yet be flexible enough to allow for cultural variations. The *ICD-11* seeks to produce more consistent diagnosis across a global, heterogeneous, multicultural, and multidisciplinary sample. The World Health Organization is particularly invested in the clinical utility of a system that functions as a tool for generating valid data-driven diagnoses. Critical to providing evidence-based health information, validated diagnoses form the basis of global statistics, health programs, and international policies.[12]

The *ICD-11* proposes a separate section on conditions related to sexual health to integrate sexual dysfunctions from the *ICD-10* sections on mental health and behavioral disorders and diseases of the genitourinary system.[13] Sexual dysfunctions and sexual pain disorders are described as syndromes associated with difficulty experiencing personally satisfying, noncoercive sexual activities regardless of the presumed cause. The proposed classifications of sexual dysfunctions will apply to both men and women (desire and orgasmic dysfunctions) unless there are distinct clinical presentations (eg, female sexual arousal dysfunction, erectile dysfunction, and ejaculatory dysfunction). Thus, desire, arousal, and orgasmic dysfunctions will be classified separately by phases and apply to both women and men in the *ICD-11*.

OVERVIEW OF FEMALE SEXUAL DISORDERS AND DIFFERENTIAL DIAGNOSIS

The human sexual response is the result of complex interactions between biological and psychosocial factors. These factors can vary between cultures, individuals, and even within the same individual depending on the time, setting, and circumstances. Different models aiming to characterize such complexities have been proposed to aid in conceptualization, diagnosis, and treatment of sexual disorders in both men and women. Perelman's[14] Sexual Tipping Point model, for example, posits that a certain threshold needs to be crossed for an individual to express sexual motivation/behavior and that many different variables can facilitate or inhibit such

Table 1
Changes in *Diagnostic and Statistical Manual of Mental Disorders* (Fifth Edition) diagnostic categories of female sexual dysfunction

DSM-IV Diagnostic Categories	*DSM-5* Diagnostic Categories
Sexual aversion disorder	Eliminated
Hypoactive sexual desire disorder FSAD	Merged into FSIAD in women
Dyspareunia Vaginismus	Merged into GPPD

expression. Other human sexual response models include the aforementioned linear model from Masters and Johnson[3] and the nonlinear model developed by Basson.[15]

There are limited data on the incidence and prevalence of FSDs. The available data differ considerably because of variations in the definitions of sexual dysfunction, different diagnostic categories used, composition of sample populations, and methods of data collection.

Incidence of FSD has been estimated to range from 25.8% to 91.0% depending on the source. A 2006 review by Hayes and colleagues[16] reported a prevalence of desire difficulties in 64% of women, arousal difficulties in 31%, orgasm difficulties in 35%, and sexual pain in 26%. A study by Burri and Spector[17] from the United Kingdom found that 5.8% of the population sampled reported current symptoms that met the criteria for an FSD diagnosis and 15.5% reported lifelong FSD. Consistent with data available from other epidemiologic studies, HSDD was the most prevalent sexual complaint. A caveat of Burri and Spector's study is that the data were derived from a sample of volunteers, with a response rate of 50%. In the PRESIDE study (Prevalence of Female Sexual Problems Associated with Distress and Determinants of Treatment Seeking) of 50,001 US women, with a 63% response rate, a prevalence of HSDD of 8.9% was reported in women aged 18 to 44 years, 12.3% in women aged 45 to 64 years, and 7.4% in women aged 65 years and older.[18] In a 5-year study following Finnish women aged 18 to 74 years, a decrease in sexual desire was identified in 45% of women: 20% among those younger than 25 years and 70% to 80% among those aged 55 to 74 years.[19] Australian and Swedish studies have reported similar findings. It is fair to say that most FSD increases with age. The most common sexual difficulty is lack of sexual interest followed by delayed orgasm (11% in Australian sample) and lack of orgasm (10%).[20,21] A consensus statement from the fourth ICSM in 2015 asserts that, across a variety of assessment methods, the prevalence of women's sexual complaints regardless of age is on the order of 40% to 50%.[22]

Multiple factors must be taken into consideration when attempting to identify a causative agent for sexual dysfunction. Medical and surgical conditions with the potential to cause sexual dysfunction can range from anatomic processes to lower urinary tract problems; endocrine disorders; malignancies, including breast and ovarian cancer; inflammatory diseases, such as fibromyalgia and rheumatoid arthritis; and neurologic conditions, such as multiple sclerosis, among others. In addition, there are a myriad of secondary (acquired) problems that can lead to sexual dysfunction, such as childbirth, hormonal changes, menopause, breastfeeding, trauma, and so forth. Psychological factors, such as depression and anxiety, are also possible causes, as are associated treatments/medications, such as antidepressants, antipsychotics, and hormonally mediated methods of birth control. Lifestyle factors, such as unhealthy diet and weight, lack of exercise, smoking, and alcohol and other substance abuse, can further contribute, as can psychosocial factors of age, education, income, and ethnicity. Other miscellaneous factors include previous history of sexual abuse, sexual orientation, type of sexual practices, negative attitudes toward sex, and negative body image.[23]

SEXUAL INTEREST AND AROUSAL DISORDERS

- HSDD is distressing low sexual desire not due to a medical or psychiatric condition or use of a substance[10] per the *DSM-IV-TR*.
- FSAD is defined as the recurrent inability to attain or maintain sufficient genital arousal despite adequate stimulation per the *DSM-IV-TR*.
- FSIAD is the result of merged HSSD and FSAD and includes both desire and arousal elements[11] per the *DSM-5*.

There are limited prevalence data available for FSIAD, including no published diagnostic validation studies or peer-reviewed literature on intervention/treatment. Thus, this diagnosis currently has almost no clinical applicability. The following information is limited to studies based on the diagnosis of HSDD, FSAD, female orgasmic disorder (FOD), and painful intercourse/penetration.

The neurobiology of desire is mediated by activation of the hypothalamus, ventral striatum, amygdala, insula, and orbitofrontal cortex[24] involving motivational and reward systems. The arousal phase of sexual response, meanwhile, correlates to a decrease in ventromedial and amygdala activation. Increases in sympathetic activity lead to enhanced vascular blood flow to the genitals resulting in physical engorgement of the vulva, clitoris, and vagina, an increase in temperature and secretions, and relaxation of the pelvic floor leading to an increase in pudendal and genitofemoral nerve conduction.[25]

Decrease in sexual desire can be attributed to specific psychosocial factors, such as physical/emotional abuse, acute life stressors, or other psychological dynamics that affect desire. Such situational causes for worsening or difficulties in sexual function should not be attributed to HSDD or FSAD. If this is the case, psychotherapeutic interventions to address the identified cause may be of benefit. Sexual dysfunction secondary to medical/psychiatric conditions or substance/medication side effects also excludes a diagnosis of HSDD and FSAD and should be addressed directly.

Current treatment modalities for disorders related to sexual desire or arousal can be broken down into 2 broad categories: hormonal treatment and nonhormonal treatment.

Hormonal treatment of HSDD and FSAD includes

- Hormone replacement with systemic or vaginal estrogen
- Androgen supplementation
- Tibolone, a selective estrogen receptor modulator (SERM)
- Ospemifene (SERM)

A 2013 Cochrane Database System review on the use of hormone replacement therapy for the purpose of improvement of sexual function in perimenopausal and postmenopausal women reported that treatment with estrogens combined with progestogens in symptomatic or early postmenopausal women led to a small to moderate benefit in sexual function in the treatment group versus control group. However, this improvement in sexual function could be largely attributed to improvements in vaginal atrophy, leading to a decrease in sexual pain and discomfort.[26]

Androgens play an important role in the treatment and management of desire disorders in women. Low levels of free and total testosterone, androstenedione, and dehydroepiandrosterone sulfate have been implicated (but not linked) to low sexual desire in women. Although topical testosterone has been studied in postmenopausal women with HSDD and intranasal testosterone has been evaluated in FOD, no androgens are currently approved by the Food and Drug Administration (FDA) for use in women. Available formulations of testosterone are dosed for men, so their use in HSDD and FSAD is strictly off label. Although anecdotal evidence and systematic studies in postmenopausal women support the safety of androgens for short-term use, long-term data on transdermal testosterone are derived only from European Union postmarketing reports.[27] The best current recommendation based on clinical trial evidence in the treatment of HSDD is for transdermal testosterone at high physiologic doses in combination with estrogen in postmenopausal women and, to a lesser degree, women in their late reproductive years.[28,29] For other populations with HSDD, such as women with premature ovarian failure or women of reproductive age, there are limited data. Among premenopausal women treated with exogenous testosterone, increased frequency of sexual activity and sexual satisfaction was observed.[30,31] Clinicians should be prepared to discuss with patients the risks associated with androgen therapy, including the androgenizing effects on a female fetus should the woman become pregnant, hirsutism, and other side effects. If supplemented, testosterone levels should be monitored periodically; if treatment with transdermal testosterone fails to show observable benefit, it should not be continued beyond 6 months.

Tibolone is a 19-nor testosterone derivative SERM available in the European Union. It is metabolized into 2 estrogenic components and a component that is both progestagenic and androgenic. The appeal of a SERM is that it is able to target different tissues selectively. Tibolone is reported to behave as an estrogen on brain, bone, and vaginal tissue, but not on breast or endometrium. Available information on its effects for women with HSDD and arousal disorders is still limited.[32–34]

Ospemifene is a nonestrogen, tissue selective estrogen receptor agonist/antagonist, or SERM, recently approved for the treatment of dyspareunia. In a randomized controlled 12-week clinical trial, ospemifene 60 mg daily was found to significantly improve female sexual function in the domains of sexual pain, arousal, and desire. The improvements did not correlate with changes in serum hormones.[35] Another study by Portman and colleagues[36] followed nonhysterectomized postmenopausal women for 52 weeks in order to assess the safety of ospemifene therapy. They concluded that daily doses of 30 mg to 60 mg yielded few treatment-emergent adverse events and demonstrated no significant endometrial changes. A meta-analysis by Cui and colleagues[37] indicated that ospemifene seems to be a safe and effective treatment of dyspareunia associated with postmenopausal vulva and vaginal atrophy.

Nonhormonal treatment of HSDD and FSAD includes

- Flibanserin
- Sildenafil
- Herbal therapy, such as ginkgo biloba extract (GBE) or ArginMax
- Eros-clitoral device
- Psychotherapy
- Bupropion

Flibanserin is a novel nonhormonal option approved by the FDA in the treatment of HSDD in premenopausal women. Its mechanism of action is through postsynaptic agonism of serotonin (5-HT)1A receptors and antagonism of 5-HT2A receptors. Flibanserin 100 mg daily at bedtime has been found to significantly improve the sexual desire domain in the Female Sexual Function Index and reduce the associated distress, as measured by the Female Sexual Distress Scale (FSDS), the two cardinal symptoms of HSDD.[38] The number of satisfying sexual events, a more downstream measure, was also significantly improved with flibanserin over placebo. Side effects of flibanserin are those commonly seen with central nervous system–active drugs and include dizziness, sedation, and nausea. A large trial in postmenopausal women with HSDD found flibanserin to be effective and well tolerated.[39] A systematic review and meta-analysis by Gao and colleagues[40] in 2015 concluded that flibanserin was effective, well tolerated, and safe in the treatment of premenopausal and postmenopausal women with HSDD.

Sildenafil is a phosphodiesterase 5 inhibitor commonly used for the treatment of erectile dysfunction in men. There is some evidence that it may play a role in the management of FSAD in women. A 2003 double-blind placebo-controlled trial found sildenafil to be effective and well tolerated in the management of FSAD in postmenopausal women.[41] All the individuals in the study were also receiving hormone replacement therapy or had protocol-specified estradiol and testosterone concentrations. There was no statistically significant improvement if the subject had FSAD and concomitant HSDD.

Basson and colleagues[42] proposed that sildenafil could potentially play a role in the female sexual arousal response based on its mechanism of action. However, a 2002 double-blind placebo-controlled clinical trial of 577 estrogenized women and 204 estrogen-deficient women with FSAD on sildenafil therapy failed to find a statistically significant effect.[42]

Conversely, a 2001 double-blind placebo-controlled study of premenopausal women demonstrated that sildenafil directly improved some symptoms of female sexual arousal disorder. In this study, the frequency of sexual fantasies and of sexual intercourse and enjoyment improved with sildenafil therapy. Of the 51 women who completed the study, 70.6% wished to continue with treatment.[43] Further studies on sildenafil for FSAD are needed.

Nutritional supplements have been proposed as potential treatments for disorders of sexual desire. GBE has been anecdotally used as herbal treatment; however, a randomized, placebo-controlled, active-comparator study found no empirical evidence to support either the short- or long-term use of GBE at a dosage of 300 mg/d.[44] Another supplement, ArginMax (containing ginseng, gingko, damiana, L-arginine, multivitamins, and minerals), was studied in a randomized controlled clinical trial of 108 premenopausal, perimenopausal, and postmenopausal women aged 22 to 73 years with complaints of low sexual desire.[45] After 4 weeks, nearly three-quarters (72%) of women treated with the supplement reported significant improvement in sexual desire and overall sexual satisfaction (68%) when compared with the placebo arm. The improvements also included increased frequency of sexual desire, reduction of vaginal dryness, increased frequency of intercourse, and satisfaction with the sexual relationship.

The Eros-Clitoral Therapy Device (Eros-CTD, NuGen, Inc) is an FDA-approved device targeting symptoms of FSAD. In a study from 2001, Wilson and colleagues[46] concluded that the Eros-CTD was safe and effective in improving symptoms of FSAD in this group of women. Further studies on the efficacy of the Eros-CTD are indicated.

Psychotherapy, specifically cognitive behavioral therapy (CBT), for HSDD and mindfulness-based group psychotherapy may have potential benefits in the treatment of FSAD. However, further systematic, controlled research is warranted.

In a multisite randomized, double-blind, placebo-controlled clinical trial by Seagraves and colleagues,[47] premenopausal women were treated with bupropion to target global idiopathic HSDD. Improvement was reported in all measures in the group receiving bupropion, including greater sexual responsiveness. The Changes in Sexual Functioning Questionnaire used in the study showed that bupropion had significant effects on increasing measures of sexual arousal, orgasm completion, and sexual satisfaction.[47]

In summary, there are a variety of therapeutic approaches that can aid in the management of desire and arousal disorders. Clinicians should strive to discover any identifiable/treatable cause of sexual dysfunction in women amenable to intervention before making a primary diagnosis of sexual dysfunction. Different approaches will be beneficial to different populations. Weighing the risks and benefits of specific treatments, such as hormonal versus nonhormonal treatment, is of paramount importance.

FEMALE ORGASMIC DISORDERS

- FOD is defined as difficulty, delayed, or inability to reach orgasm during sexual activity and includes reduced frequency and/or intensity of experience of orgasm.
- Orgasmic dysfunction–associated distress is a necessary criterion for diagnosis.
- FOD is the second most prevalent sexual disorder in women.[48]

Orgasm is defined as a sensation of intense pleasure resulting in a physiologic reaction and sensations of well-being and contentment. It is typically accompanied by an altered state of consciousness, involuntary rhythmic contractions of pelvic striated vaginal musculature, uterine and anal contractions, and a reduction of sexually induced vasocongestion eventually leading to a release of tension and positive feelings. Women are able to attain orgasm through a variety of methods, most commonly direct clitoral and vaginal stimulation but also and not infrequently reported through breast/nipple stimulation, mental imagery, fantasy and hypnosis, and may occur during rapid eye movement sleep.[49,50]

Brain changes with orgasm have been documented via functional MRI and PET, demonstrating increased activation in the paraventricular nucleus of the hypothalamus, periaqueductal gray region of the midbrain, hippocampus, and cerebellum in women with spinal-cord injury.[51]

Genetic factors have been associated with the ability to achieve orgasm during intercourse and masturbation with a hereditability of 34% and 45%, respectively.[52] Single nucleotide polymorphisms in glutamatergic receptor genes have been associated with difficulty attaining orgasm.[53]

Psychological aspects, including body image, self-esteem, relationship conflict, and preoccupation with genital appearance and perceived odor, can negatively affect a woman's ability to relax.[54,55] These difficulties can lead women to perceive their lack of orgasm as a failure, engendering feelings of shame, guilt, depression, distress, and anxiety, reinforcing negative beliefs about one's ability and perpetuating orgasmic difficulties.[56] Other factors that can potentially affect a woman's ability to attain orgasm include past history of sexual abuse, low score in emotional intelligence questionnaires, and other personality traits, such as emotional instability, introversion, and not being open to new experiences.[57]

In a 2016 study of 866 women in the general population, 48% of women had difficulty with orgasm during partnered sex at least half the time, with younger women having more problems than older women.[58] Among those women with orgasmic difficulties, 57% voiced moderate to severe associated distress. Almost half admitted to moderate to severe problems with arousal. Findings from the National Social and Health Life Survey reported a prevalence of FOD of 24%, without accounting for associated distress, in a random sample of 1749 US women.[59] In the aforementioned PRESIDE study, 21% of 31,581 women aged 18 years and older reported having problems with orgasm, and 4.6% of those also reported significant personal distress using the FSDS.[18] Thus, conservative estimates of the prevalence of FOD are approximately 5%. Given the high degree of distress and frustration FOD can cause, goals of treatment should enable women with this condition to achieve sexual satisfaction, lessen or resolve impediments to orgasm, and experience improvements in quality of life.[60]

Current treatment options for FOD are limited. Management includes CBT focused on reducing anxiety-provoking thoughts and cognitions that cause sexual difficulties, sensate focus aimed at increasing intimacy and trust, Kegel exercises, bibliotherapy, communications skills training, and direct clitoral stimulation.[61]

A 2007 study of tibolone in FOD showed improved orgasm in postmenopausal women using more than one metric.[62] Enhanced arousal with agents such as bupropion, sildenafil, granisetron, estrogen, and testosterone has proven to be of limited efficacy in treatment of FOD. Intranasal oxytocin and bremelanotide have also been postulated as potential agents to study in the treatment of anorgasmia; however, data supporting clinical use for this application are lacking.

FEMALE SEXUAL PAIN DISORDERS

GPPD is a new diagnostic category in the *DSM-5* that merges the previous diagnosis of vaginismus and dyspareunia into a single sexual pain disorder associated with vaginal penetration. As with FSIAD, no field trials or diagnostic validity studies are yet available with this new diagnosis. It may be that at least 2 distinct diagnostic entities with different etiologic factors and distinct treatments have been subsumed under this single diagnosis.

Other classification systems include the ISSVD and ICSM (**Table 2**).

The estimated prevalence for dyspareunia ranges from 6.5% to 45.0% in older women to 14% to 35% in younger women. Estimates for prevalence of vaginismus are harder to find in the literature. Current available data indicate a prevalence of 7.8% for vulvar pain and 1.0% to 6.0% for vaginismus.[63] Exact prevalence estimates are difficult to obtain because of the high variability between studies secondary to discrepancies in classification systems, different definitions, and variable survey methods.

As is the case with other FSDs, GPPD is a cause of low levels of sexual satisfaction, reduced well-being, and relationship difficulties.[64] Some significant differences in response to sexual stimuli have been identified in women with vaginismus/dyspareunia and women without pain during intercourse. Women with vaginismus report negative cognitions and beliefs about sex and have a negative/avoidant response to sexual stimuli, erotic films and other erotic material.[65] This type of avoidance/fear reaction can be triggered by psychological stimuli, physical stimulation, or a combination of both.

There is no single etiologic factor associated with GPDD, hence, the importance of history taking and physical examination. It is critical to obtain a detailed description of onset, severity, and symptom perception. A thorough history should include level of anxiety; effect of sexual positions; pain during manual, phallic, or tampon insertion; menopausal status; alleviating factors; and onset and constancy of symptoms. Consider taking partner's report when indicated.

A comprehensive pain and psychosocial assessment is of utmost importance in providing diagnostic clarity. **Table 3** summarizes minimum elements in assessment recommended by the ICSM's 2015 expert consensus.

Table 2
Clinical features of genital pain disorders

Condition	Clinical Feature
Dyspareunia	Genital pain associated with sexual intercourse
Vaginismus	Involuntary spasm/tension of perineal and levator muscles making penetration difficult/not possible; intense fear of pain
Vestibulodynia	Severe pain on touch or attempted vaginal entry within vestibule
Vulvodynia	Chronic neuropathic-like pain in vulvar area that can persist independent of physical contact

Table 3
Pain and psychosocial assessment

Pain	Pain quality, time of onset, temporal pattern, duration, location, elicitors, intensity
Musculoskeletal history	Surgeries, injury, fall to the lumbar-pelvic-hip region, tailbone, and sacrum
Bowel and bladder	Habits and function history
Sexuality	Desire, arousal, orgasm, frequency, satisfaction, sexual practice, and distress
Psychological	Thoughts, emotions, behaviors, couple interactions (avoidance, conflict, hypervigilance, partner responses, and self-efficacy) Childhood trauma Current romantic relationship
Comorbidities	Other medical and mental health conditions
Treatment	Previous treatment attempts, interventions, and outcomes
Questionnaires	Standardized self-report questionnaires, such as Female Sexual Function Index

Data from Goldstein AT, Pukall CF, Brown C, et al. Vulvodynia: assessment and treatment. J Sex Med 2016;13(4):572–90.

The use of rating scales allows clinicians to establish a baseline and track progress. Multiple pain rating scales are available to measure different aspects covered in **Table 3**. Some examples of available tools are summarized in **Table 4**.

It is important to remember that although screening tools are useful in many clinical settings, characterizing physical real-time pain through a physical examination is essential and can provide invaluable information. Hence, patients should be referred to a qualified professional who can perform a complete gynecologic examination and who is mindful and knowledgeable on the topic. A cotton swab test is the standard test for the diagnosis of provoked vulvodynia.[71] Other examinations to characterize pain and identify cause might include the tampon test, a modified one finger method manual examination, and use of a pediatric-sized speculum.[72]

The clinician should look for a variety of possible anatomic and functional causes, which can be divided into irritative, anatomic, and infectious.

Irritative causes include poor lubrication, atrophic vaginitis, vulvar dermatoses, and vulvodynia. Anatomic causes include endometriosis, fibroids, bladder or uterine prolapse, gynecologic malignancy, and scar tissue from previous surgical procedures or episiotomy. Infectious causes are varied but include sexually transmitted infections

Table 4
Genital pain screening and evaluation tools

McGill Pain Questionnaire[67]	78 Adjectives to Describe Types of Pain
Pain Catastrophizing Scale[68]	Psychological predictor of pain and disability
Painful Intercourse Self-efficacy Scale[69]	20 items with 3 subscales assessing women's perceived ability to carry out sexual activities
Vaginal Penetration Cognition Questionnaire[70]	40-item questionnaire with 5 cognition subscales: control, positive, catastrophic and pain, self-image, and genital incompatibility
Vulvar Pain Functional Questionnaire	11 questions assessing for provoked and unprovoked vulvar pain

(STIs), such as gonorrhea, chlamydia, and others that can cause pelvic inflammatory disease, as well as non-STIs, such as chlamydial vulvovaginitis.

Irritative causes of vaginal pain can be treated with the use of lubricants and moisturizers. Some nonhormonal options include water-based, silicon-based and mineral oil–based lubricants. Mineral oil–based products should not be used if condoms are being used for protection from STIs or for contraception, as oil-based products can potentially weaken the integrity of the latex. If other irritative causes of pain and pruritus, such as lichen planus or lichen sclerosus, are suspected, an evaluation by a dermatologist is indicated.

Other treatment options include hormonal topical products and systemic estrogen to address atrophic vaginitis in postmenopausal women. Topical hormones are preferred to systemic hormones because of the lower risk profile. It is important to be aware that topical doses great than 50 μg can be absorbed systemically and are, hence, not considered low-dose vaginal treatment. Some options include estradiol vaginal tablets 10 μg, estradiol cream, estradiol ring, and conjugated estrogen cream. Experts in the field state that treatment with topical estrogens can still be considered in women with atrophic vaginitis who have had breast cancer. Starting in February 2016, the American College of Obstetricians and Gynecologists supports the use of vaginal estrogen in women with a history of estrogen-dependent breast cancer.[73]

Oral preparation of ospemifene can be used for the management of vaginal atrophy and painful intercourse in postmenopausal women.[35] This selective estrogen reuptake modulator has been shown to be effective at doses of 30 mg to 60 mg daily.[74] Currently, the FDA recommends use of concomitant progestin, but there are not enough data to substantiate this recommendation since ospemifene is not known to affect the endometrial lining. Some potential cautions include the unknown safety profile in women after breast cancer diagnosis. There is also a reported increased risk of thrombotic events.

Once all organic causes have been excluded, a diagnosis of GPDD can be made. For vulvodynia, topical anesthetic preparations and steroids are not recommended for long-term use. Experts from the Fourth International Consultation on Sexual Medicine recommend the following management: psychological interventions, pelvic floor physical therapy with or without biofeedback when the pelvic floor is found to be restricted or overactive, and vestibulectomy in cases of provoked vestibulodynia. A multidisciplinary approach is strongly recommended.[66] Surgical management should be considered if conservative approaches have failed. Surgical vulvar vestibulectomy has shown good success rates, including symptom improvement in women with provoked vestibular pain. Other treatments, such as capsaicin cream and botulinum toxin, are not recommended as the primary line of treatment but can be considered as second-line options. There is no evidence to support the use of tricyclic antidepressants (TCA) in the management of vulvodynia, and no recommendations regarding TCAs exist for GPPD.[75]

Male partner's responses to the sexual pain are also prognostic factors that can be either detrimental or beneficial to sexual functioning. Partner coping styles that are either manifested as solicitous, providing attention and sympathy, or negative, manifesting as hostility and frustration, are associated with further deterioration and avoidance of sexual activity. Partner's facilitative response is a positive factor, encouraging healthier sexual activity and adaptive coping.[76]

When physical causes have been ruled out, attention to possible somatization fear/anxiety psychogenic factors in vaginismus may be of benefit, especially in women who rate high in alexithymia. Fear has been reported as a factor exacerbating phobic attitudes toward sexual stimuli by Melles and colleagues.[77,78] Therapeutic modalities for vaginismus include sex therapy and systematic desensitization. Therapist-aided exposure treatment was effective in reducing subjective fear of sexual penetration stimuli and led to more global positive affective associations with sexual stimuli. However, a 2012 Cochrane Database review showed no clinical or statistical difference between systematic desensitization and wait-list control, systematic desensitization combined with group therapy or in vitro (with women under instruction by the therapist) desensitization, in the treatment of vaginismus.[79]

SECONDARY CAUSES OF SEXUAL DYSFUNCTION

An important *DSM* exclusion criterion in the diagnosis of primary FSD is that symptoms not be due to a medical or psychiatric condition or a substance (medication, alcohol, illicit drugs, and so forth). The most common identifiable cause of sexual dysfunction in women is depression and treatment with antidepressant medications. Depression is a well-known cause of a generalized decrease in interest, motivation and enjoyment in life, with specific effects on sexual interest, activity, and satisfaction. Sexual function and depression have a bidirectional relationship with depression accounting for a 50% to 70% increased risk of developing sexual dysfunction, and sexual dysfunction increasing the risk of developing depression by 130% to 210%.[80] Before starting treatment with an antidepressant, assessment of baseline functioning using a standard metric such as the Changes in Sexual Functioning Questionnaire or the Arizona Sexual Experiences Scale plus patient preference may inform choice of antidepressant therapy. Clinicians should consider prescribing an antidepressant that is less likely to cause sexual side effects, and patients should made aware of all potential side effects. Patients are often reluctant to spontaneously report sexual side effects due to fear of feeling judged or discomfort with a taboo subject. By normalizing and setting the right expectations, a channel of communication between patient and doctor can be established to address these important concerns. Assessment at follow-up to monitor sexual functioning related to treatment of depression and onset or increased sexual dysfunction due to medication side effect should be performed. The principles described are applicable to other conditions and substances.

Although depression itself can be an important cause of sexual dysfunction, treatment with antidepressant medications has also been reported to cause impairment in sexual function in 25% to 80% of people taking these medications, with a class effect of serotonin reuptake inhibitors having the most negative effects on sexual desire and function.[81] Medications with other mechanisms of action (eg, bupropion, mirtazapine, vortioxetine, vilazodone) or different delivery systems (eg, transdermal selegiline) seem to be associated with better sexual functioning.[82]

Of note, 5% to 10% of people taking antidepressants will experience spontaneous amelioration of sexual symptoms after being on an antidepressant for 4 to 6 months.[83] However, about 90% of those affected by antidepressants will continue to experience sexual dysfunction, even if depressive symptoms remit.

Multiple randomized controlled clinical trials have found the addition of sustained-release bupropion can ameliorate symptoms related to decreased sexual desire in women with selective serotonin reuptake inhibitor (SSRI)–induced sexual dysfunction.[47] A Cochrane Database Systematic review identified 5 quality studies confirming a reduction of sexual side effects related to SSRI treatment when bupropion was added.[84] Buspirone similarly has also been found to be an effective antidote/adjunctive treatment to antidepressant-associated sexual dysfunction.[85] A clinical trial of sildenafil therapy to

Table 5
Selective studies of antidepressants with assessment of effects on sexual function

Study	Study Design	Effect on Sexual Dysfunction
Serretti & Chiesa,[81] 2009	Meta-analysis	• SSRIs (sertraline, citalopram, paroxetine, escitalopram, fluoxetine), SNRIs (venlafaxine, duloxetine), TCA (imipramine, phenelzine), and fluvoxamine associated with more sexual dysfunction compared with placebo • No statistically significant difference between placebo and agomelatine, amineptine, bupropion, moclobemide, mirtazapine, and nefazodone
Ozmenler Karlidere et al,[88] 2008	Open-label study	• Reduction in Psychotropic-Related Sexual Dysfunction Questionnaire scores (PRSexDQ-SALSEX) (indicating improved sexual function) from augmentation with mirtazapine
Clayton, Kornstein et al,[89] 2007	Double-blind, placebo-controlled study	• Higher incidence of sexual dysfunction with escitalopram compared with duloxetine and placebo
Clayton, Croft et al,[90] 2006	Randomized, double-blind, placebo-controlled study	• Bupropion XL similar to placebo and more favorable sexual function profile compared with escitalopram
Thase et al,[91] 2006	Double-blind, multicenter study	• Bupropion XL less negative effect on sexual function compared with venlafaxine XR
Kennedy, Fulton et al,[92] 2006	Randomized, double-blind controlled study	• Worsened sexual dysfunction in patients on paroxetine compared with bupropion SR
Clayton, Pradko et al,[93] 2002	Multicenter, cross-sectional, observational study	• Increased rate of sexual dysfunction with SSRIs (citalopram, paroxetine, sertraline and fluoxetine) and SNRI (venlafaxine XR) compared with bupropion XL

Abbreviation: SNRI, serotonin-norepinephrine reuptake inhibitor.

target symptoms of SSRI-induced sexual dysfunction reported some improvement in arousal and orgasmic ability in women.[86]

Of note, improved sexual function in women taking SSRIs may result if sexual activity occurs within 30 minutes of cardiovascular training.[87] The positive effects of exercise did not seem to carry over if sexual activity occurred outside that time frame (**Table 5**).

SUMMARY

Female sexual function is affected by a complex variety and balance of physical, psychosocial, hormonal, and genetic factors. A clear, unified, and accessible classification system is needed to standardize diagnosis and treatment of individuals experiencing sexual dysfunction. Ideally, such a system could be used by both researchers and clinicians alike to provide a reliable database for global health statistics and help guide the development of interventions and implementation of important health policies.

An integrative approach that encompasses experts in different fields of medicine is crucial to further our understanding of the causes of FSD. Advancement toward a more precise nomenclature and classification system of FSD will facilitate better diagnosis, research, and development and selection of treatments options, all of which will ultimately lead to superior care for women with sexual dysfunction.

REFERENCES

1. Wright JJ, O'Connor KM. Female sexual dysfunction. Med Clin North Am 2015;99: 607–28.
2. Sungur MZ, Gunduz A. A comparison of DSM-IV-TR and DSM-5 definitions for sexual dysfunctions: critiques and challenges. J Sex Med 2014;11(2):364–73.
3. Masters W, Johnson V. Human sexual response. Boston: Little, Brown and Company; 1966.
4. Sand M, Fisher WA. Women's endorsement of models of female sexual response: the nurses' sexuality study. J Sex Med 2007;4(3):708–19.
5. Giles KR, McCabe MP. Conceptualizing women's sexual function: linear vs. circular models of sexual response. J Sex Med 2009;6(10):2761–71.
6. Giraldi A, Kristensen E, Sand M. Endorsement of models describing response of men and women with a sexual partner: an online survey in a population sample of Danish adults ages 20-65 years. J Sex Med 2015;12(1):116–28.
7. Sarin S, Amsel RM, Binik YM. Disentangling desire and arousal: a classificatory conundrum. Arch Sex Behav 2013;42(6):1079–100.
8. DeRogatis LR, Clayton AH, Rosen RC, et al. Should sexual desire and arousal disorders in women be merged? Arch Sex Behav 2011;40(2):217–9.
9. Segraves RT, Balon R, Clayton A. Proposal for changes in diagnostic criteria for sexual dysfunctions. J Sex Med 2007;4:567–80.
10. American Psychiatric Association. Diagnostic and statistical manual of mental disorders: DSM- IV-TR. Washington, DC: American Psychiatric Publishing; 2000.
11. American Psychiatric Association. Diagnostic and statistical manual of mental disorders. 5th edition. Arlington (VA): American Psychiatric Publishing; 2013.
12. First MB, Reed GM, Hyman SE, et al. The development of the ICD-11 clinical descriptions and diagnostic guidelines for mental and behavioural disorders. World Psychiatry 2015;14:82–90.
13. Reed GM, Drescher J, Krueger RB, et al. Disorders related to sexuality and gender identity in the ICD-11: revising the ICD-10 classification based on current scientific evidence, best clinical practices, and human rights considerations. World Psychiatry 2016;15:205–21.
14. Perelman MA. The sexual tipping point: a mind/body model for sexual medicine. J Sex Med 2009;6(3):629–32.
15. Basson R. Female sexual response: the role of drugs in the management of sexual dysfunction. Obstet Gynecol 2001;98(2):350–3.
16. Hayes RD, Bennett CM, Fairley CK, et al. What can prevalence studies tell us about female sexual difficulty and dysfunction? J Sex Med 2006;3(4):589–95.
17. Burri A, Spector T. Recent and lifelong sexual dysfunction in female UK population sample: prevalence and risk factors. J Sex Med 2001;8:2420–30.
18. Shifren JL, Monz BU, Russo PA, et al. Sexual problems and distress in United States women: prevalence and correlates. Obstet Gynecol 2008;112:970–8.

19. Kontula O, Haavio-Mannila E. Sexual pleasures. Enhancement of sex life in Finland. 1971-1992. Dartmouth (NH): Aldershot Publishing; 1995.
20. Smith AMA, Lyons A, Ferris JA, et al. Incidence and persistence/recurrence of women's sexual difficulties: findings from the Australian Longitudinal Study of Health and Relationships. J Sex Marital Ther 2012;38:378–93.
21. Fugl-Meyer KS. Sexual disabilities and sexual problems. In: Fugl-Meyer KS, editor. Sex in Sweden. (pp 199). Stockholm (Sweden): Swedish National Institute of Health; 2000.
22. McCabe MP, Sharlip ID, Atalla E, et al. Definitions of sexual dysfunctions in women and men: a consensus statement from the fourth International Consultation on Sexual Medicine 2015. J Sex Med 2016;13:135–43.
23. Khajehei M, Doherty M, Tilley M. An update on sexual function and dysfunction in women. Arch Womens Ment Health 2015;18:423–33.
24. Kingsberg SA, Clayton AH, Pfaus JG. The female sexual response: current models, neurobiological underpinnings and agents currently approved or under investigation for the treatment of hypoactive sexual desire disorder. CNS Drugs 2015;29(11):915–33.
25. Schultz WW, van Andel P, Sabeli I, et al. Magnetic resonance imaging of male and female genitals during coitus and female sexual arousal. BMJ 1999;319: 1596–600.
26. Nastri CO, Lara LA, Ferriani RA, et al. Hormone therapy for sexual function in perimenopausal and postmenopausal women. Cochrane Database Syst Rev 2013;(6):CD009672.
27. Shifren JL, Davis SR, Moreau M, et al. Testosterone patch for the treatment of hypoactive sexual desire disorder in naturally menopausal women: results from the INTIMATE NM1 Study. Menopause 2006;13:770.
28. North American Menopause Society. The role of testosterone therapy in postmenopausal women: position statement of the North American Menopause Society. Menopause 2005;12:496.
29. Davis SR, Worsley R, Miller KK, et al. Androgens and female sexual function and dysfunction- findings from the fourth International Consultation of Sexual Medicine. J Sex Med 2016;13(2):168–78.
30. Fooladi E, Davis SR. An update on the pharmacological management of female sexual dysfunction. Expert Opin Pharmacother 2012;13(15):2131–42.
31. Goldstat R, Briganti E, Tran J, et al. Transdermal testosterone therapy improves well-being, mood, and sexual function in premenopausal women. Menopause 2003;10:390–8.
32. Cayan F, Dilek U, Pata O, et al. Comparison of the effects of hormone therapy regimens, oral and vaginal estradiol, estradiol + drospirenone and tibolone, on sexual function in healthy postmenopausal women. J Sex Med 2008;5:132–8.
33. Wu MH, Pan HA, Wang ST, et al. Quality of life and sexuality changes in postmenopausal women receiving tibolone therapy. Climacteric 2001;4:314.
34. Nijland EA, Weijmar Schultz WC, Nathorst-Boös J, et al, LISA study investigators. Tibolone and transdermal E2/NETA for the treatment of female sexual dysfunction in naturally menopausal women: results of a randomized active-controlled trial. J Sex Med 2008;5(3):646–56.
35. Constantine G, Graham S, Portman DJ, et al. Female sexual function improved with ospemifene in postmenopausal women with vulvar and vaginal atrophy: results of a randomized, placebo-controlled trial. Climacteric 2015;18(2):226–32.

36. Portman DJ, Bachman GA, Simon JA. Ospemifene, a novel selective estrogen receptor modulator for treating dyspareunia associated with postmenopausal vulvar and vaginal atrophy. Menopause 2013;20(6):623–30.
37. Cui Y, Zong H, Yan H, et al. Ospemifene, a novel selective estrogen receptor modulator for treating dyspareunia associated with postmenopausal vulvar and vaginal atrophy. J Sex Med 2014;11(2):487–97.
38. Vallejos X, Wu C. Flibanserin: a novel, nonhormonal agent for the treatment of hypoactive sexual desire disorder in premenopausal women. J Pharm Pract 2016. [Epub ahead of print].
39. Simon JA, Kingsberg SA, Shumel B, et al. Efficacy and safety of flibanserin in postmenopausal women with hypoactive sexual desire disorder: results of the SNOWDROP trial. Menopause 2014;21:633–40.
40. Gao Z, Yang D, Yu L, et al. Efficacy and safety of flibanserin in women with hypoactive sexual desire disorder: a systematic review and meta-analysis. J Sex Med 2015;12:2095–104.
41. Berman JR, Berman LA, Toler SM, et al. Safety and efficacy of sildenafil citrate for the treatment of female sexual arousal disorder: a double-blind, placebo controlled study. J Urol 2003;170(6 Pt 1):2333–8.
42. Basson R, McInnes R, Smith MD, et al. Efficacy and safety of sildenafil citrate in women with sexual dysfunction associated with female sexual arousal disorder. J Womens Health Gend Based Med 2002;11(4):367–77.
43. Caruso S, Intelisano G, Lupo L, et al. Premenopausal women affected by sexual arousal disorder treated with sildenafil: a double-blind, cross-over, placebo-controlled study. BJOG 2001;108(6):623–8.
44. Meston CM, Rellini AH, Telch MJ. Short- and long-term effects of Ginkgo biloba extract on sexual dysfunction in women. Arch Sex Behav 2008;37(4):530–47.
45. Ito TY, Polan ML, Whipple B, et al. The enhancement of female sexual function with ArginMax, a nutritional supplement, among women differing in menopausal status. J Sex Marital Ther 2006;32(5):369–78.
46. Wilson SK, Delk JR, Billups KL. Treating symptoms of female sexual arousal disorder with the Eros-Clitoral Therapy Device. J Gend Specif Med 2001;4(2):54–8.
47. Seagraves RT, Clayton A, Croft H, et al. Bupropion sustained release for the treatment of hypoactive sexual desire disorder in premenopausal women. J Clin Psychopharmacol 2004;24(3):339–42.
48. Kinsberg SA, Tkachenko N, Lucas J, et al. Characterization of orgasmic difficulties by women: focus group evaluation. J Sex Med 2013;10:2242–50.
49. Fisher C, Cohen HD, Schiavi RC, et al. Patterns of female arousal during sleep and waking: vaginal thermoconductance studies. Arch Sex Behav 1983;12(2):97–122.
50. Wells BL. Nocturnal orgasms: females' perception of a "normal" sexual experience. J Sex Res 1983;22:412–37.
51. Komisaruk BR, Whipple B. Functional MRI of the brain during orgasm in women. Annu Rev Sex Res 2005;16:62–86.
52. Dunn KM, Cherkas LF, Spector TD. Genetic influences on variation in female orgasmic function: a twin study. Biol Lett 2005;1(3):260–3.
53. Perlis RH, Laje G, Smoller JW, et al. Genetic and clinical predictors of sexual dysfunction in citalopram-treated depressed patients. Neuropsychopharmacology 2009;34(7):1819–28.
54. Braun V, Wilkinson S. Socio-cultural representations of the vagina. J Reprod Infant Psychol 2001;18(1):17–32.

55. Schick VR, Calabrese SK, Rima BN, et al. Genital appearance dissatisfaction: implications for women's genital image self-consciousness, sexual esteem, sexual satisfaction, and sexual risk. Psychol Women Q 2010;34(3):394–404.
56. Birnbaum GE. The meaning of heterosexual intercourse among women with female orgasmic disorder. Arch Sex Behav 2003;32:61–71.
57. Burri AV, Cherkas LM, Spector TD. Emotional intelligence and its association with orgasmic frequency in women. J Sex Med 2009;6(7):1930–7.
58. Rowland DL, Kolba TN. Understanding orgasmic difficulty in women. J Sex Med 2016;13(8):1246–54.
59. Laumann EO, Paik A, Rosen RC. Sexual dysfunction in the United States: prevalence and predictors. JAMA 1999;281(6):537–44.
60. Redelman M. A general look at female orgasm and anorgasmia. Sex Health 2006; 3(3):143–53.
61. Meston CM, Hull E, Levin RJ, et al. Disorders of orgasm in women. In: Lue TF, Basson R, Rosen R, et al, editors. Sexual dysfunctions in men and women. Paris: Health Publications; 2004 (Summary of Committee).
62. Kamenov ZA, Todorova MK, Christov VG. Effect of tibolone on sexual function in late postmenopausal women. Folia Med (Plovdiv) 2007;49(1–2):41–8.
63. Jacques JD, et al. Women's sexual pain disorders. J Sex Med 2010;7:616–31.
64. Simonelli C, EWluteri S, Petrucelli F, et al. Female sexual pain disorders: dyspareunia and vaginismus. Curr Opin Psychiatry 2014;27:406–12.
65. Cherner RA, Reissing ED. A psychophysiological investigation of sexual arousal in women with lifelong vaginismus. J Sex Med 2013;42:1605–14.
66. Goldstein AT, Pukall CF, Brown C, et al. Vulvodynia: assessment and treatment. J Sex Med 2016;13(4):572–90.
67. Melzack R. The McGill Pain Questionnaire: major properties and scoring methods. Pain 1975;1:277–99.
68. Sullivan MJL, Biship S, Pivik J. The pain catastrophizing scale: development and validation. Psychol Assess 1995;7:524–32.
69. Desrochers G, Bergeron S, Khalife S, et al. Fear avoidance and self-efficacy in relation to measure perceived self-efficacy in people with arthritis. Semin Arthritis Rheum 1989;32(1):37–44.
70. Hummel-Berry K, Wallave K, Herman H. Reliability and validity of the vulvar functional status questionnaire (VQ). J Womens Health Phys Therap 2007;31(3): 1605–14.
71. Friederich EG. Vulvar vestibulitis syndrome. J Reprod Med 1987;32(2):110.
72. Foster D, Kotox M, Huang L, et al. The tampon test for vulvodynia treatment outcomes research reliability construct validity, and responsiveness. Obstet Gynecol 2009;113(4):825–32.
73. Committee Opinion No. 659. American College of Obstetricians and Gynecologists. The use of vaginal estrogen in women with a history of estrogen-dependent breast cancer. Obstet Gynecol 2016;127:e93–6.
74. Bachmann GA, Komi JO, Ospemifene Study Group. Ospemifene effectively treats vulvovaginal atrophy in postmenopausal women: results from a pivotal phase 3 study. Menopause 2010;17(3):480–6.
75. Leo RJ, Dewani S. A systematic review of the utility of antidepressant pharmacotherapy in the treatment of vulvodynia pain. J Sex Med 2013;10:2497–505.
76. Rosen NO, Bergeron S, Sadikaj G, et al. Impact of male partner responses on sexual function in women with vulvodynia and their partners - a dyadic daily experience study. Health Psychol 2014;33:823–31.

77. Melles RJ, Ter Kuile MM, Dewitte M, et al. Automatic and deliberate affective associations with sexual stimuli in women with lifelong vaginismus before and after therapist aided exposure treatment. J Sex Med 2014;11:786–99.
78. Ter Kuile MM, Melles RJ, Tuijnman-Raasveld CC, et al. Therapist aided exposure for women with lifelong vaginismus: mediators of treatment outcome: a randomized waiting list control trial. J Sex Med 2015;12(8):1807–19.
79. Melnik T, Hawton K, McGuire H. Interventions for vaginismus. Cochrane Database Syst Rev 2012;(12):CD001760.
80. Atlantis E, Sullivan T. Bidirectional association between depression and sexual dysfunction: a systematic review and meta-analysis. J Sex Med 2012;9(6): 1497–507.
81. Serretti A, Chiesa A. Treatment-emergent sexual dysfunction related to antidepressants: a meta-analysis. J Clin Psychopharmacol 2009;29(3):259–66.
82. Clayton AH, Alkis AR, Parik NH, et al. Sexual dysfunction due to psychotropic medications. Psychiatr Clin North Am 2016;39(3):427–63.
83. Clayton AH, Montejo AL. Major depressive disorder, antidepressants, and sexual dysfunction. J Clin Psychiatry 2006;67(Suppl 6):33–7.
84. Taylor MJ, Rudkin L, Bullemor-Day P, et al. Strategies for managing sexual dysfunction induced by antidepressant medication. Cochrane Database Syst Rev 2013;(5):CD003382.
85. Landen M, Eriksson E, Agren H, et al. Effect of buspirone on sexual dysfunction in depressed patients treated with selective serotonin reuptake inhibitors. J Clin Psychopharmacol 1999;19(3):268–71.
86. Nunberg HG, Hensley PL, Heiman JR, et al. Sildenafil treatment of women with antidepressant-associated sexual dysfunction: a randomized controlled trial. JAMA 2008;300(4):395–404.
87. Lorenz TA, Meston CM. Exercise improves sexual function in women taking antidepressants: results from a randomized crossover trial. Depress Anxiety 2014; 31(3):188–95.
88. Ozmenler NK, Karlidere T, Bozkurt A, et al. Mirtazapine augmentation in depressed patients with sexual dysfunction due to selective serotonin reuptake inhibitors. Hum Psychopharmacol 2008;23(4):321–6.
89. Clayton A, Kornstein S, Prakash A, et al. Changes in sexual functioning associated with duloxetine, escitalopram, and placebo in the treatment of patients with major depressive disorder. J Sex Med 2007;4(4 Pt 1):917–29.
90. Clayton AH, Croft HA, Horrigan JP, et al. Bupropion extended release compared with escitalopram: effects on sexual functioning and antidepressant efficacy in 2 randomized, double-blind, placebo-controlled studies. J Clin Psychiatry 2006; 67(5):736–46.
91. Thase ME, Clayton AH, Haight BR, et al. A double-blind comparison between bupropion XL and venlafaxine XR: sexual functioning, antidepressant efficacy, and tolerability. J Clin Psychopharmacology 2006;26(5):482–8.
92. Kennedy SH, Fulton KA, Bagby RM, et al. Sexual function during bupropion or paroxetine treatment of major depressive disorder. Can J Psychiatry 2006; 51(4):234–42.
93. Clayton AH, Pradko JF, Croft HA, et al. Prevalence of sexual dysfunction among newer antidepressants. J Clin Psychiatry 2002;63(4):357–66.

Women and Addiction: An Update

Nassima Ait-Daoud, MD[a,*], Derek Blevins, MD[a], Surbhi Khanna, MD[a], Sana Sharma, MD[a], Christopher P. Holstege, MD[b], Pooja Amin, BS, MD[c]

KEYWORDS

• Women • Substance abuse • Alcohol • Opioids • College female students

KEY POINTS

- Substance abuse among women is on the rise.
- Women use and respond to drugs differently from men.
- Biological, social, cultural, and environmental factors have an impact on a woman's substance use and recovery difficulties.
- Comprehensive treatment programs catering to the needs of women are required for a better outcome.

INTRODUCTION

Women and men often use alcohol and drugs for different reasons and respond to them differently. Research has identified unique characteristics related to hormones, fertility, pregnancy, breastfeeding, and menopause that can impact women's progression from use to addiction and struggles with recovery. In addition, there are culturally defined roles for men and women that further impact the differences seen in the 2 genders and affect the way they seek help. In 2003, an estimated 5.9% of women aged 18 or older met criteria for abuse of or dependence on alcohol or an illicit drug in the past year.[1] This number has increased, as now women are the fastest-growing segment of substance users in the United States. This increase in prevalence of women with

This is an update of an article that first appeared in the *Psychiatric Clinics of North America*, Volume 40, Issue 2, June 2017.

Disclosure of Commercial and Noncommercial Interests: The authors do not have any commercial financial interests to disclose.

[a] Department of Psychiatry and Neurobehavioral Sciences, University of Virginia, PO Box 800623, Charlottesville, VA 22908, USA; [b] Division of Medical Toxicology, Department of Emergency Medicine, University of Virginia, PO Box 800774, Charlottesville, VA 22908-0774, USA; [c] Center for Leading Edge Addiction Research (CLEAR) Department of Psychiatry and Neurobehavioral Sciences, University of Virginia, 560 Ray C Hunt Drive, Charlottesville, VA 22903-2981, USA

* Corresponding author.

E-mail address: NAT7B@hscmail.mcc.virginia.edu

Med Clin N Am 103 (2019) 699–711

http://dx.doi.org/10.1016/j.mcna.2019.03.002 medical.theclinics.com

alcohol or drug (AOD) use has unique serious adverse health consequences, given that women experience a more rapid progression of their addiction than men.[2]

AOD use disorder is an isolating problem for women of all ages. Many women with such disorders hide their addiction, as they fear that seeking help while pregnant or afterward could have legal or social ramifications. Women with AOD disorders tend to isolate more and are more likely to experience partner violence and abuse.[3]

ALCOHOL USE IN WOMEN

According to the National Institute on Alcohol Abuse and Alcoholism (NIAAA), men may be at risk for alcohol-related problems if their alcohol consumption exceeds 14 standard drinks per week or 4 drinks per day, and women 7 standard drinks per week or 3 drinks per day.[4] Women absorb and metabolize alcohol differently from men. They have higher blood alcohol concentrations after consuming the same amount of alcohol because they have a smaller amount of total body water and lower activity of the alcohol metabolizing enzyme, alcohol dehydrogenase (ADH) in the stomach, causing a larger proportion of the ingested alcohol to be absorbed. Therefore, women are more susceptible to the negative health consequences of alcohol, such as alcoholic liver disease, heart problems,[5] and brain damage.[6]

Alcohol's deleterious effect on the overall cognitive function is well documented. Even mild-to-moderate drinking can adversely affect cognitive functioning, including mental activities that involve acquiring, storing, retrieving, and using information.[7] Persistent cognitive impairment can interfere with learning and academic achievement in youth with an established pattern of chronic heavy drinking.[8] There is additional evidence suggesting that women may be more vulnerable to alcohol-induced neurodegeneration than men, with worse performance on tests of recall and psychomotor speed.[9]

Alcohol-induced liver damage is dose-dependent, making women at higher risk for developing alcoholic liver disease over a shorter period and more likely to die from cirrhosis when compared with men.[10,11] Another possible mechanism of alcohol-induced liver damage is the effects of estrogen on endotoxin and lipid peroxidation, both of which promote alcoholic liver injury.[12]

Sex hormones are affected by consumption of alcohol with a differential effect based on age. One study found that estrogen levels were depressed among adolescent girls ages 12 to 18 for as long as 2 weeks after drinking moderately,[13] presumably by affecting luteinizing hormone release hormone production and therefore interfering with the hypothalamus-pituitary axis regulation of estrogen release. In female rats, puberty was markedly delayed when the rats were given ethanol.[14–16] These findings suggest the possibility that alcohol may alter the reproduction maturity that occurs during puberty and may negatively affect growth spurt and normal progression of puberty in human female adolescents. In premenopausal women, alcohol intake has been associated with higher concentrations of estradiol, estrone, and testosterone, as well as decreases in follicle-stimulating hormone.[17,18] This increase in endogenous estrogen is presumably caused by alcohol-induced suppression of the normal nocturnal rise in melatonin, which in turn would increase the release of sex hormones from the ovaries. Increase in endogenous estrogen is believed to raise the risk for breast cancer in this age group.[17,18] This mechanism is thought to explain the relationship of alcohol to the risk of lobular and hormone receptor–positive breast cancer, but not on other types of breast cancer.[19] Even in postmenopausal women who are on estrogen replacement therapy, there is also evidence suggesting that alcohol consumption may increase blood estradiol levels, and therefore may increase their risk of breast cancer.[20–22] Studies conducted did not, however, account for dietary variations, such as amount of folate intake, which could affect outcomes.[23] Alcohol also may increase risk for cancer through its negative effect on the immune system. It impairs chemotaxis or the ability of white blood cells to migrate to sites of injury or infection[24] and alters production of macrophages and cytokines and causes an elevation in immunosuppressive glucocorticoids.[25]

Maternal alcohol use during pregnancy contributes to a range of developmental, cognitive, and behavioral problems in exposed children, including hyperactivity and attention problems, learning and memory deficits, and problems with social and emotional development. These developmental problems and disabilities are grouped under fetal alcohol spectrum disorder (FASD). Drinking threshold for the development of FASD has not been adequately identified.[26] Because no one knows how much alcohol is safe during pregnancy, the US Surgeon General issued an advisory warning pregnant women and women who might become pregnant to abstain from any alcohol use.

Although light-to-moderate drinking among women has been reported to be associated with reduced risks of some cardiovascular problems, the same levels of drinking are also associated with increased risks of breast cancer and liver function problems. With chronic heavy drinking, women are at increased risk for osteoporosis-related complications[27] and cognitive deficits.[28]

WOMEN AND THE OPIOID EPIDEMIC

Although we have experienced a rise in both prescription and nonprescription opioid use in the United States in the past 2 decades, women have been disproportionately affected by the "opioid epidemic," with different diagnostic and treatment considerations compared with men. One of the most staggering effects of the surge in opioid misuse is the dramatic increase in opioid-related overdoses, accounting for nearly 30,000 of the 47,000 lethal drug overdoses that occurred in 2014.[29] From 1999 through 2010, 48,000 women died of overdoses from prescription opioids, representing a 400% increase in prescription opioid-related deaths compared with a 237% increase among men.[30] Furthermore, past-year heroin use nearly doubled between 2005 and 2012,[31] with 4 of 5 new heroin users reporting initial narcotics exposure through prescription opioids.[32] The increase in heroin use among women resulted in a tripling of the number of women dying from heroin overdose in the 3 years between 2010 and 2013.[33] This disproportionate outcome for women is consistent with past studies that have indicated that women progress to problematic substance use more rapidly than men after using smaller amounts of a substance over a shorter period, despite the lower overall prevalence of substance use disorders among women compared with men.[34]

One factor likely playing a significant role is that women are more likely to have chronic pain, for which they are prescribed opioids at higher doses and longer-term use compared with men. Furthermore, women are more likely to "doctor shop" to obtain controlled substances, an issue that may be intertwined with the higher prevalence of chronic pain.[35] Interestingly, emergency department data indicate that women in the 25 to 54 years age group are the most likely to present for prescription painkiller misuse or abuse,[33] rather than elderly women with age-related chronic pain. There are also recent preclinical data to suggest some role for female sex hormones in the development or maintenance of problematic opioid use, with female rats consistently reducing heroin self-administration by 70% when estradiol and progesterone levels are high during proestrus.[36] However, prior preclinical studies have had mixed results regarding the role of sex hormones in opioid self-administration.[37,38] These issues raise important points regarding the prevention, recognition, and the treatment of opioid use disorders in women.

Family responsibilities and finances may differentially limit women from obtaining appropriate treatment for an opioid use disorder, particularly with methadone maintenance therapy requiring daily visits.[39] Finally, women may be treated differently based on their fertility status, given that opioids are known to cause neonatal abstinence syndrome (NAS) and various other birth defects.[40] In a New York Medicaid population, the proportion of women who received opioid prescriptions was highest among women with an indication of contraceptive use or infertility (27%), and lowest during the prenatal period for women who had a live birth (9.5%).[41] Interestingly, 17% of women with no documented use of contraceptive measure or infertility received opioid prescriptions, indicating a need to better ascertain women's gynecologic status before starting treatment.[40]

Both chronic pain and "doctor shopping" reinforce the importance of state-run prescription drug monitoring programs to prevent or identify problematic use among both men and women. Once an opioid use disorder is identified, methadone and buprenorphine (BUP) remain the standard medication-assisted treatment, regardless of gender, but issues specific to women, like the lack of child care, may prevent them from seeking or being able to maintain opioid agonist treatment, which requires daily or weekly appointments.[33]

Unlike methadone treatment, which must be performed at a highly structured clinic, BUP is the first medication to treat opioid dependency that can be prescribed in a physician's office. BUP and BUP/Naloxone combination are medications approved by the Food and Drug Administration for medication-assisted treatment of opioid use disorder. BUP is a partial μ-opioid receptor agonist, which competes with other opioid agents at the μ opioid sites.[42] BUP's opioid effects increase with each dose until a moderate dose is reached, after which there is a "ceiling effect" on both the euphoric and respiratory depressive properties; therefore, lowering the risk of misuse, overdose, and side effects. To further decrease its abuse liability, naloxone is added. However, naloxone has no to minimal absorption when the combination is taken sublingually. If injected, snorted, or ingested, naloxone is absorbed, releasing its antagonist action at the opioid receptor level, therefore blocking any opioid effect.

The standard treatment for opioid dependency in pregnant women is methadone. A National Institute of Drug Abuse (NIDA)-sponsored clinical trial, the Maternal Opioid Treatment: Human Experimental Research (MOTHER) study, found BUP to be equally safe compared with methadone in the treatment of opioid dependence among pregnant women, with the added benefit of a reduced intensity of NAS compared with infants born to women who received methadone.[43] One limitation with the use of BUP in pregnant women is switching them from a pure agonist to a partial agonist, which may cause discomfort and withdrawal symptoms at the beginning of the treatment. BUP may therefore be a good option for pregnant women who are new to treatment and are in active opioid withdrawal or who become pregnant while on this medication. If a patient is on methadone maintenance and stable, however, she should remain on methadone through the pregnancy.

COCAINE USE IN WOMEN

In animal research, female rats were found to be more sensitive to the drug-reinforcing effects and exhibited higher levels of motivation for cocaine self-administration than male rats.[44] Similarly, when men and women were given cocaine in a laboratory study, women consistently scored higher than men on mental and physical well-being after receiving cocaine.[45] Sex hormones, mainly estrogen, play a significant role in alcohol and drug-dependence acquisition by enhancing drug-seeking behavior,[46] potentially impacting women's pattern of drug use and treatment response. Long-term cocaine use suppresses neuroendocrine systems and sex hormones, leading to a disruption of the estrous cycle, and therefore, fertility problems.[47,48]

When pregnant, often women who are considered regular users of cocaine, do not discontinue cocaine use and consistently use larger amounts of other drugs, including tobacco, alcohol, and marijuana compared with pregnant women who do not use cocaine.[49,50] The usual pattern of cocaine use among pregnant women and others includes periods of binges followed by forced abstinence and withdrawal. This leads to increases in the use of other drugs of abuse in an effort to cope with the withdrawal symptoms and cravings. In a study conducted by Mbah and colleagues,[51] women who abused cocaine were found to be 58% more likely to have placenta-associated syndrome (PAS) when compared with women who did not (odds ratio = 1.48, 95% confidence interval: 1.33–1.66). Maternal PAS includes abnormal conditions during pregnancy associated with placental dysfunction, such as pre-eclampsia, eclampsia, gestational hypertension, placental infarction, placental abruption, and oligohydramnios. These adverse events have negative pregnancy and fetal outcomes, including mortality.

Cocaine abusers in general are at an increased risk for contracting human immunodeficiency virus (HIV) and other infectious diseases. This risk stems not only from sharing contaminated needles and other drug paraphernalia, but also from engaging in risky behaviors as a result of drug intoxication.[52] In addition, research indicates that HIV-infected women progress to AIDS with just half the amount of virus circulating in their bloodstream as compared with men.[53] It is not clear what causes this gender disparity, but according to the Centers for Disease Control and Prevention, drug abuse accounts for a greater percentage of cases of HIV infection among women than men.[54] This may be caused by the greater impact of AOD-induced suppression of the immune system seen in women, allowing for more rapid viral replication and disease progression.

MARIJUANA USE IN WOMEN

Marijuana is an increasingly popular drug in the United States, especially among youth, due to easy accessibility and perceived benefits, such as relaxation and stress relief. According to the latest National Survey on Drug Use and Health report, an estimated 22.2 million Americans aged 12 years or older are current marijuana users.[55] Most marijuana users in the United States are between the ages of 18 and 29 years (56.4%), white (70.9%), and male (66.3%).[56]

Sex differences between male and female marijuana users have been studied. Men use cannabis more frequently and more excessively than women; however, women are twice as likely as men to initiate use after age 30.[57] There is a significant association between heavy marijuana use and development of suicidality in men, but not in women.[58] On the other hand, there is a significant association between past suicidality and initiation of cannabis use in women.[55]

Female marijuana users demonstrate greater craving in response to drug cues than men.[59] Women also report greater subjective positive effects from marijuana than men despite no differences in levels of intoxication.[60] This may increase the risk of women developing cannabis use disorder earlier than men who use the same amount of marijuana. Women also differ from men in several aspects of marijuana use, including reasons for use, triggers, response to treatment, and vulnerability to relapse.[56]

Several states in the United States have now legalized marijuana, and physicians must be aware that marijuana is the most commonly used illicit drug during pregnancy.[61] Women using marijuana at least weekly during pregnancy are at a significant high risk of low birth weight, stillbirth, and preterm deliveries.[62] Women using marijuana might also be using tobacco and other illicit substances, which act as confounding factors. According to Ko and colleagues,[63] 10.9% of pregnant women and 14% of nonpregnant women of reproductive age in the United States reported past-year marijuana use in 2007 to 2012. Despite these high numbers, our current understanding of marijuana use during pregnancy and its long-term effects on the fetus remains poor.[64] More research is needed in this field because of the growing number of pregnant women seeking help for marijuana use during pregnancy and lactation.[58]

Clinicians should be aware of women of all ages using marijuana and should be able to provide patient education and specific resources, including comprehensive treatment for use of other substances.[59] Women are more likely than men to maintain a social network, speak more freely about marijuana use, and remain abstinent after treatment, but are also more likely to relapse in response to negative emotions or interpersonal problems.[56] A higher dose of cannabis is associated with a significant increase in prevalence of mood and anxiety disorders in women with cannabis use disorder compared with those without cannabis use disorder,[53] and this must be addressed appropriately.

ALCOHOL AND SUBSTANCE USE AMONG FEMALE COLLEGE STUDENTS

College students make up one of the largest groups of drug abusers nationwide.[65,66] As students are facing the high demands of coursework, part-time jobs, internships, peer pressure, and social obligations, many turn to drugs and alcohol as a way to cope. Historically, women experienced a greater shame about drinking and intoxication than men, but it appears that among younger women, this stigma is slowly fading. Although male students are generally more likely to report drug use and abuse, female students are still more likely to drink and to binge. Women are drinking more and frequently than they did in the past. In 2013, 59.4% of full-time college students, ages 18 to 22 drank alcohol in the past month compared with 50.6% of other persons of the same age, with 12.7% being engaged in heavy drinking (5 or more drinks on an occasion on 5 or more occasions per month) in the past month compared with 9.3% of persons of the same age not attending college.[67] According to data from a survey of almost 18,000 college students across the United States, approximately 1 in 3 female students engage in binge drinking with the rate of binge drinking in all-female colleges doubling between 1993 and 2001.[68] Binge drinking is defined by NIAAA as "a pattern of drinking that brings blood alcohol concentration levels to 0.08 g/dL. This typically occurs after 4 drinks for women in about 2 hours." Female college students are at higher risk of being assaulted or raped as a consequence of heavy drinking, with 97,000 students between the ages of 18 and 24 reporting having experienced alcohol-related sexual assault or date rape and 696,000 students reporting being assaulted by another student who has been drinking.[69]

SUBSTANCE ABUSE AND PREGNANCY

It is well established that the use of illicit drugs during pregnancy poses a significant risk to the developing fetus. An NIDA-funded study found that newborns whose mothers abused methamphetamine during pregnancy showed higher rates of growth restriction at birth.[51] Indeed, methamphetamine and other stimulant use in pregnancy endangers the health of the mother and increases the risk of low birth weight and infants small for gestational age, and such use may increase the risk of subsequent neurodevelopmental problems in childhood. Similarly, infants born to mothers who abuse cocaine during pregnancy are often premature, have low birth weights and smaller head circumferences, and are shorter in length than infants born to mothers who do not abuse cocaine. Prenatal nicotine exposure is harmful to both the mother and the fetus. It alters neurologic development in experimental animals and may increase the risk for neurologic conditions in humans.[70] There is a positive association between maternal smoking during pregnancy and sudden infant death syndrome[71]; prenatal nicotine exposure may also alter auditory response and how sounds are interpreted by the auditory cortex.[72,73] Even the use of marijuana during pregnancy may result in problems with neurologic development. Most marijuana-exposed infants show signs of an altered response to visual stimuli, increased tremulousness, and a high-pitched cry, which may stem from problems with neurologic development.[74]

It is important to consider other factors that are often closely linked with alcohol and drug abuse in women, such as neglect of their children, exposure to violence, poor socioeconomic conditions, and poor maternal health. Additionally, there is evidence that children who have been exposed to drugs prenatally are more likely to develop substance abuse problems and other mental health issues, and are more likely to suffer from cognitive impairment, memory problems, and attention deficit difficulties.[68,75,76]

EVALUATION

According to the Substance Abuse and Mental Health Services Administration,[77] when evaluating women using alcohol or illicit drugs, clinicians must consider trauma history, pregnancy, and resulting intrauterine effects of AOD use and identify barriers to accessing health care. Specific characteristics in women may prevent them from seeking treatment, including their complex roles of mother, partner, and caregiver, and fear of losing custody of children who are under their care if the AOD problem is admitted. Women are more likely to experience mental health problems as a result of their AOD use. In women with co-occurring disorders, 55% to 99% have experienced trauma from abuse and tend to engage in self-destructive behaviors.[78]

Women prefer to seek help for their substance abuse in mental health facilities rather than drug treatment centers, as it is easier for them to discuss their psychological distress and symptoms of mood and anxiety than acknowledging their AOD use during the first visit. Women tend to enter treatment sooner after they develop substance dependence than men,[79] but require more accommodations to stay in treatment, such as child care resources and transportation. Integrated, trauma-informed treatment services will increase the success of their recovery. Although active outreach interventions work better for men, women respond better to an office-based setting and they feel safer discussing sensitive matters away from pressure from family or drug dealers.[80]

Screening for alcohol disorders in primary care can vary from using a standardized questionnaire, such as the CAGE questionnaire (felt need to *cut back*, *annoyed* by critics, *guilt* about drinking, and *eye-opening* morning drink)[81,82] or other available instruments (see the NIAAA Web site for a full listing http://pubs.niaaa.nih.gov/publications/AssessingAlcohol/selfreport.htm). Clinicians who may not have time for a lengthy assessment can use the single alcohol screening question (SASQ), "When was the last time you had more than 4 drinks in 1 day?" This SASQ has a sensitivity and specificity of 0.86 in identifying current alcohol use disorders.[83,84]

In prenatal-care settings, the T-ACE (*Tolerance to alcohol, annoyed* by critics, need to *cut back,* and *eye-opening morning drink*), a 4-item questionnaire based on the

CAGE, can identify alcohol consumption in pregnant women. It has been tested in a wide variety of obstetric practices and has proven to be a valuable and efficient tool for identifying an alcohol use disorder.[85,86] Also, simply asking about a woman's drinking pattern before she becomes pregnant may help solicit more accurate information on her current drinking.

Similarly, a general question about lifetime use of any illicit substances can orient the health care provider to more focused questions. For a more structured interview, the health care provider can use the NIDA-modified "Alcohol, Smoking and Substance Involvement Screening Test" (ASSIST) questionnaire that scores each substance endorsed, identifies the risk level, and from there orients the interviewer to the type of intervention needed from simple advice to referral.[87,88]

SUMMARY

In general, women begin using drugs at lower doses than men, but drug use escalates more rapidly to addiction, and women face a greater risk for negative health consequences and relapse after abstinence. Women are more vulnerable than men to the effects of alcohol. Even in small amounts, alcohol may increase the risk of breast cancer, osteoporosis, liver disease, hormonal imbalance, and issues with fertility. On college campuses, female students who drink heavily on occasion are at higher risk for assaults, unwanted sexual advances, and unplanned and unsafe sex. The significant role of trauma and abuse in women with AOD use disorder is often not addressed in most treatment programs, as they are tailored mostly for men. It is important that women seek help in office-based settings, preferably in primary, prenatal care, or mental health clinics. Greater awareness by the health care community of the specific issues that women with AOD use disorders face is needed to help reduce the disparities in treatment availability and acceptability across genders.

REFERENCES

1. Office of Applied Studies, Substance Abuse and Mental Health Services Administration (SAMHSA). NSDUH Report August 5, 2005: Substance Abuse and Dependence among Women. Available at: http://www.oas.samhsa.gov/2k5/women/women.htm. Accessed September 3, 2010.
2. Greenfield SF, Pettinati HM, O'Malley S, et al. Gender differences in alcohol treatment: an analysis of outcome from the COMBINE study. Alcohol Clin Exp Res 2010;34(10):1803–12.
3. Kumpfer KL. Links between prevention and treatment for drug-abusing women and their children. In: National Institute on Drug Abuse, Drug Addiction Research and the Health of Women, editors. Rockville (MD): US Department of Health and Human Services, National Institutes of Health; 1998. p. 565–72.
4. National Institutes of Health: The Office of Research on Women's Health, Office of the Director, the National Institute on Alcohol Abuse and Alcoholism. Alcohol: A Women's Health Issue. Available at: http://pubs.niaaa.nih.gov/publications/brochurewomen/women.htm. Accessed September 3, 2010.
5. Urbano-Márquez A, Estruch R, Fernández-Solá J, et al. The greater risk of alcoholic cardiomyopathy and myopathy in women compared with men. JAMA 1995;274(2):149–54.
6. Nixon SJ. Cognitive deficits in alcoholic women. Alcohol Health Res World 1994;18(3):228–32.

7. Evert DL, Oscar-Berman M. Alcohol-related cognitive impairments: an overview of how alcoholism may affect the workings of the brain. Alcohol Health Res World 1995;19(2):89–96.
8. Giancola PR, Moss HB. Executive cognitive functioning in alcohol use disorder, recent developments in alcoholism, the consequences of alcoholism, vol. 14. New York: Plenum Pressrs; 1998. p. 227–51.
9. Acker C. Performance of female alcoholics on neuropsychological testing. Alcohol 1985;20(4):379–86.
10. Pequignot G, Tuyns AJ. Greater risk of ascitic cirrhosis in females in relation to alcohol consumption. Int J Epidemiol 1984;13(1):53–7.
11. Hall P. Factors influencing individual susceptibility to alcoholic liver disease. In: Hall P, editor. Alcoholic liver disease: pathology and pathogenesis. 2nd edition. London: Edward Arnold; 1995. p. 299–316.
12. Kono H, Wheeler MD, Rusyn I, et al. Gender differences in early alcohol-induced liver injury: role of CD14, NF-kappaB, and TNF-Alpha. Am J Physiol Gastrointest Liver Physiol 2000;278(4):652–61.
13. Block GD, Yamamoto ME, Mallick A, et al. Effects on pubertal hormones by ethanol abuse in adolescents. Alcohol Clin Exp Res 1993;17(2):505.
14. Dees WL, Skelley CW, Hiney JK, et al. Actions of ethanol on hypothalamic and pituitary hormones in prepubertal female rats. Alcohol 1990;7(1):21–5.
15. Skelly CW, Dees WL. Effects of ethanol during the onset of female puberty. Neuroendocrinology 1990;51(1):64–9.
16. Dees WL, Dissen GA, Hiney JK, et al. Alcohol ingestion inhibits the increased secretion of puberty-related hormones in the developing female rhesus monkey. Endocrinology 2000;141(4):1325–31.
17. Reichman M, Judd J, Longcope C, et al. Effects of alcohol consumption on plasma and urinary hormone concentrations in pre-menopausal women. J Natl Cancer Inst 1993;85(9):722–7.
18. Stevens R, Davis S, Mirick D, et al. Alcohol consumption and urinary concentration of 6-sulfatoxymelatonin in healthy women. Epidemiology 2000;11(6):660–5.
19. Li CI, Chlebowski RT, Freiberg M, et al. Alcohol consumption and risk of postmenopausal breast cancer by subtype: the women's health initiative observational study. J Natl Cancer Inst 2010;102(18):1422–31.
20. Tseng M, Longnecker M. Alcohol, hormones, and postmenopausal women. Alcohol Health Res World 1998;22(3):185–9.
21. Purohit V. Moderate alcohol consumption and estrogen levels in postmenopausal women: a review. Alcohol Clin Exp Res 1998;22(5):994–7.
22. Gronbaek M, Nielsen NR. Interactions between intakes of alcohol and postmenopausal hormones on risk of breast cancer. Int J Cancer 2008;122(5):1109–13.
23. Sellers TA, Kushi LH, Cerhan JR, et al. Dietary folate intake, alcohol, and risk of breast cancer in a prospective study of postmenopausal women. Epidemiology 2001;12(4):420–8.
24. Bautista AP. Free radicals, chemokines, and cell injury in HIV-1 and SIV infections and alcoholic hepatitis. Free Radic Biol Med 2001;31(12):1527–32.
25. Messingham KA, Kovacs EJ. Influence of alcohol and gender on immune response. Alcohol Res Health 2002;26(4):257–63.
26. Jacobson SW, Jacobson JL. Effects of prenatal alcohol exposure on child development. Alcohol Res Health 2002;26(4):282–6.
27. Sampson HW. Alcohol and other factors affecting osteoporosis risk in women. Alcohol Res Health 2002;26(4):292–8.

28. Sullivan EV, Fama R, Rosenbloom MJ, et al. A profile of neuropsychological deficits in alcoholic women. Neuropsychology 2002;16(1):74.
29. Centers for Disease Control and Prevention, National Center for Health Statistics, National Vital Statistics System, et al. Number and age-adjusted rates of drug-poisoning deaths involving opioid analgesics and heroin: United States, 2000–2014. Atlanta (GA): Center for Disease Control and Prevention; 2015. Available at: http://www.cdc.gov/nchs/data/health_policy/AADR_drug_poisoning_involving_OA_Heroin_US_2000. 2014.pdf.2015.
30. Center for Disease Control and Prevention. Prescription painkiller overdoses: a growing epidemic, especially among women. Atlanta (GA): Centers for Disease Control and Prevention; 2013. Available at: http://www.cdc.gov/vitalsigns/prescriptionpainkilleroverdoses/index.html.
31. Substance Abuse and Mental Health Services Administration, Results from the 2012 national survey on drug use and health: summary of national findings, NSDUH Series H-46, HHS Publication no. (SMA) 13-4795. Rockville (MD): Substance Abuse and Mental Health Services Administration.
32. Jones CM. Heroin use and heroin use risk behaviors among nonmedical users of prescription opioid pain relievers - United States, 2002-2004 and 2008-2010. Drug Alcohol Depend 2013;132(1–2):95–100.
33. Hedegaard H, Chen LH, Warner M. Drug-poisoning deaths involving heroin: United States, 2000–2013. NCHS Data Brief, no 190. Hyattsville (MD): National Center for Health Statistics; 2015. Available at: http://www.cdc.gov/nchs/data/databriefs/db190.htm.
34. NIDA. Substance Use in Women. Available at: https://www.drugabuse.gov/publications/drugfacts/substance-use-in-women. Accessed February 23, 2017.
35. Center for Disease Control and Prevention. Prescription painkiller overdoses: a growing epidemic, especially among women. Atlanta (GA): Centers for Disease Control and Prevention; 2013. Available at: http://www.cdc.gov/vitalsigns/prescriptionpainkilleroverdoses/index.html. Accessed February 23, 2017.
36. Lacy RT, Strickland JC, Feinstein MA, et al. The effects of sex, estrous cycle, and social contact on cocaine and heroin self-administration in rats. Psychopharmacology 2016;233(17):3201–10.
37. Roth ME, Casimir AG, Carroll ME. Influence of estrogen in the acquisition of intravenously self-administered heroin in female rats. Pharmacol Biochem Behav 2002;72:313–8.
38. Stewart J, Woodside B, Shaham Y. Ovarian hormones do not affect the initiation and maintenance of intravenous self-administration of heroin in the female rate. Psychobiology 1996;24:154–9.
39. Green CA. Gender and use of substance abuse treatment services. Available at: http://pubs.niaaa.nih.gov/publications/arh291/55-62.htm. Accessed February 23, 2017.
40. Broussard CS, Rasmussen SA, Reefhuis J, et al. Maternal treatment with opioid analgesics and risk for birth defects. Am J Obstet Gynecol 2011;204(4):314.e1–e11.
41. Gallagher BK, Shin Y, Roohan P. Opioid prescriptions among women of reproductive age enrolled in Medicaid — New York, 2008–2013. Morb Mortal Wkly Rep 2016;65:415–7.
42. Center for Substance Abuse Treatment. Clinical guideline for the use of buprenorphine in the treatment of opioid addiction. Treatment Improvement Protocol (TIP) Series 40. DHHS publication no. (SMA) 04-3939. Rockville (MD): Substance Abuse and Mental Health Services Administration; 2004.

43. Jones HE, Kaltenbach K, Heil SH, et al. Neonatal abstinence syndrome after methadone or buprenorphine exposure. N Engl J Med 2010;363:2320–31.
44. Lynch WJ, Roth ME, Carroll ME. Biological basis of sex differences in drug abuse: preclinical and clinical studies. Psychopharmacology (Berl) 2002;164(2):121–37.
45. Nich C, McCance-Katz EF, Petrakis IL, et al. Sex differences in cocaine-dependent individuals' response to disulfiram treatment. Addict Behav 2004; 29(6):1123–8.
46. Carroll ME, Lynch WJ, Roth ME, et al. Sex and estrogen influence drug abuse. Trends Pharmacol Sci 2004;25(5):273–9.
47. Mello NK. Cocaine abuse and reproductive function in women. Available at: http://archives.drugabuse.gov/PDF/DARHW/131-150_Mello.pdf. Accessed September 3, 2010.
48. Teoh SK, Mello NK, Mendelson JH. Effects of drugs of abuse on reproductive function in women and pregnancy. In: Watson R, editor. Addictive behaviors in women. Totowa (NJ): Humana Press; 1994. p. 437–73.
49. Minnes S, Singer LT, Humphrey-Wall R, et al. Psychosocial and behavioral factors related to the post-partum placements of infants born to cocaine-using women. Child Abuse Negl 2008;32:353–66.
50. Singer LT, Arendt R, Minnes M, et al. Increased psychological distress in post-partum, cocaine using mothers. J Subst Abuse 1995;7:165–74.
51. Mbah AK, Alio AP, Fombo DW, et al. Association between cocaine abuse in pregnancy and placenta-associated syndromes using propensity score matching approach. Early Hum Dev 2012;88(6):333–7.
52. Strathdee SA, Galai N, Safaiean M, et al. Sex differences in risk factors for HIV seroconversion among injection drug users: a 10-year perspective. Arch Intern Med 2001;161(10):1281–8.
53. Farzadegan H, Hoover DR, Astemborski J, et al. Sex differences in HIV-1 viral load and progression to AIDS. Lancet 1998;352(9139):1510–4.
54. Smith LM, LaGasse LL, Derauf C, et al. The infant development, environment, and lifestyle study: effects of prenatal methamphetamine exposure, polydrug exposure, and poverty on intrauterine growth. Pediatrics 2006;118(3):1149–59.
55. Center for Behavioral Health Statistics and Quality. Behavioral health trends in the United States: results from the 2014 National Survey on Drug Use and Health (HHS Publication No. SMA 15-4927, NSDUH Series H-50); 2015. Available at: http://www.samhsa.gov/data/. Accessed February 23, 2017.
56. Lev-Ran S, Imtiaz S, Taylor BJ, et al. Gender differences in health-related quality of life among cannabis users: results from the national epidemiologic survey on alcohol and related conditions. Drug Alcohol Depend 2012;123(1–3):190–200.
57. Cuttler C, Mischley LK, Sexton M. Sex differences in cannabis use and effects: a cross-sectional survey of cannabis users. Cannabis and Cannabinoid Research 2016;1(1):166–75.
58. Shalit N, Shoval G, Shlosberg D, et al. The association between cannabis use and suicidality among men and women: a population-based longitudinal study. J Affect Disord 2016;205:216–24.
59. Fattore L. Considering gender in cannabinoid research: a step towards personalized treatment of marijuana addicts. Drug Test Anal 2013;5(1):57–61.
60. Haney M, Cooper ZD. Investigation of sex-dependent effects of cannabis in daily cannabis smokers. Drug and Alcohol Dependence 2014;136:85–91.
61. Martin CE, Longinaker N, Mark K, et al. Recent trends in treatment admissions for marijuana use during pregnancy. J Addict Med 2015;9(2):99–104.

62. Conner SN, Bedell V, Lipsey K, et al. Maternal marijuana use and adverse neonatal outcomes. Obstet Gynecol 2016;128(4):713–23.
63. Ko JY, Farr SL, Tong VT, et al. Prevalence and patterns of marijuana use among pregnant and nonpregnant women of reproductive age. Am J Obstet Gynecol 2015;213(2):201.e1-10.
64. Volkow ND, Baler RD, Compton WM, et al. Adverse health effects of marijuana use. N Engl J Med 2014;370(23):2219–27.
65. Johnston LD, O'Malley PM, Miech R, et al. Monitoring the future national survey results on drug use, 1975-2015: overview, key findings on adolescent drug use. Ann Arbor (MI): Institute for Social Research, The University of Michigan; 2016.
66. NIDA. College-age & young adults. Available at: https://www.drugabuse.gov/related-topics/college-age-young-adults. Accessed February 23, 2017.
67. SAMHSA, National Survey on Drug use and Health (NSDUH). Table 6.88B—Alcohol use in the Past Month among Persons Aged 18 to 22, by College Enrollment Status and Demographic Characteristics: Percentages, 2012 and 2013. Available at: http://www.samhsa.gov/data/sites/default/files/NSDUH-DetTabs2013/NSDUH-DetTabs2013.htm#tab6.88b. Accessed February 23, 2017.
68. Wechsler H, Kuh G, Davenport AE. Fraternities, sororities and binge drinking: results from a National Study of American Colleges. NASPA J 2009;46(3):395–416.
69. Hingson R, Heeren T, Winter M, et al. Magnitude of alcohol-related mortality and morbidity among U.S. College students ages 18–24: changes from 1998 to 2001. Annu Rev Public Health 2005;26:259–79.
70. Rende EK, Blood-Siegfried J. The long-term effects of prenatal nicotine exposure on neurologic development. J Midwifery Womens Health 2010;55(2):143–52.
71. Sundell H, Milerad J. Nicotine exposure and the risk of SIDS. Acta Paediatr Suppl 1993;82(389):70–2.
72. Liang K, Poytress BS, Weinberger NM, et al. Nicotinic modulation of tone-evoked responses in auditory cortex reflects the strength of prior auditory learning. Neurobiol Learn Mem 2008;90(1):138–46.
73. Liang K, Poytress BS, Chen Y, et al. Neonatal nicotine exposure impairs nicotinic enhancement of central auditory processing and auditory learning in adult rats. Eur J Neurosci 2006;24(3):857–66.
74. Smith AM, Fried PA. A literature review of the consequences of prenatal marihuana exposure: an emerging theme of a deficiency in aspects of executive function. Neurotoxicol Teratol 2001;23(1):1–11.
75. Broening HW, Morford LL, Inman-Wood SL, et al. 3,4-Methylenedioxymethamphetamine (ecstasy)-induced learning and memory impairments depend on the age of exposure during early development. J Neurosci 2001;21(9):3228–35.
76. Singer LT, Arendt R, Minnes S, et al. Cognitive and motor outcomes of cocaine-exposed infants. JAMA 2002;287(15):1952–60.
77. Broening HW, Morford LL, Inman-Wood SL, et al. 3,4-Methylenedioxymethamphetamine (ecstasy)-induced learning and memory impairments depend on the age of exposure during early development. J Neurosci 2001;21:3228–35.
78. Covington SS, Burke C, Keaton S, et al. Evaluation of a trauma-informed and gender-responsive intervention for women in drug treatment. J Psychoactive Drugs 2008;40(Suppl 5):387–98.
79. Grella CE. From generic to gender-responsive treatment: changes in social policies, treatment services, and outcomes of women in substance abuse treatment. J Psychoactive Drugs 2008;(Suppl 5):327–43.

80. Trotter RT, Bowen AM, Baldwin JA, et al. Efficacy of network-based HIV/AIDS risk-reduction programs in midsized towns in the United States. J Drug Issues 1996;26(3):591–605.
81. Ewing JA. Detecting alcoholism, the CAGE questionnaire. JAMA 1984;252(14):1905–7.
82. Fiellin DA, Reid MC, O'Connor PG. Screening for alcohol problems in primary care: a systematic review. Arch Intern Med 2000;160(13):1977–89.
83. Vinson DC, Williams RH. Validation of a single screening question for problem drinking. J Fam Pract 2001;50(4):307–12.
84. Taj N, Devera-Sales A, Vinson DC. Screening for problem drinking: does a single question work? J Fam Pract 1998;46(4):328–35.
85. Sokol RJ, Martier SS, Ager JW, T-ACE Questions. Practical prenatal detection of risk-drinking. Am J Obstet Gynecol 1989;160(4):863–8.
86. Chang G, Wilkins-Haug L, Berman S, et al. Alcohol use in pregnancy: improving identification. Obstet Gynecol 1998;91(6):892–8.
87. Humeniuk R, Dennington V, Ali R. The effectiveness of a brief intervention for illicit drugs linked to the alcohol, smoking and substance involvement screening test (ASSIST) in primary health care settings: a technical report of phase III findings of the WHO ASSIST randomized controlled trial. Geneva (Switzerland): World Health Organization; 2008.
88. National Institute on Drug Abuse (NIDA). NM Assist Screening for Drug use in General Medical Setting: National Institute on Drug Abuse. Available at: http://ww1.drugabuse.gov/nmassist/. Accessed September 3, 2010.

Dementia in Women

Todd M. Derreberry, MD, Suzanne Holroyd, MD*

KEYWORDS

- Dementia • Women • Caregiver burden • Alzheimer's dementia
- Women as caregivers

KEY POINTS

- Dementia is a growing problem in women worldwide, overall occurring more often in women than men.
- Considering specific types of dementia, Alzheimer disease occurs more often in women, whereas other less common dementias, such as vascular dementia, dementia of Lewy body type, and Parkinson disease dementia do not.
- Women may survive longer with Alzheimer dementia but may have a more rapid and severe course in the associated cognitive decline.
- Women are more likely to serve as a caregiver to someone with dementia, thus are at increased risk of caregiver stress.

Dementia is a significant health problem worldwide and it affects women disproportionately compared with men. This is both in the numbers of women diagnosed with dementia, as well as caregiver burden. Increasing knowledge of dementia in women is crucial for health care providers of all specialties to more appropriately meet this important health care need.

EPIDEMIOLOGY OF DEMENTIA

For both genders, the world population is becoming older. Internationally, by 2050, the world population of adults older than 60 is projected to increase by 1.25 billion.[1] This is true also for the United States, as according to the US Census Bureau the number of older adults (age 65 and older) is expected to increase from 43.1 to 83.7 million between 2012 and 2050.[2] As advancing age is a major risk factor for dementia, the prevalence of dementia is also increasing with the larger population of older adults. A 2013 meta-analysis estimated a doubling of the prevalence of dementia every 5 to 7 years.[1]

This article originally appeared in the *Psychiatric Clinics of North America*, Volume 40, Issue 2, June 2017.
No commercial or financial conflicts of interest.
Department of Psychiatry and Behavioral Medicine, Joan C. Edwards School of Medicine, Marshall University, 1115 20th Street, Suite 201, Huntington, WV 25703, USA
* Corresponding author.
E-mail address: holroyds@marshall.edu

Med Clin N Am 103 (2019) 713–721
http://dx.doi.org/10.1016/j.mcna.2019.02.004 **medical.theclinics.com**

Alzheimer's Disease International estimated that global numbers of those effected by dementia would rise from 44.35 million in 2013 to 135.46 million by 2050.[3] In addition to the health burden of the rising prevalence of dementia, there is the related vast financial burden. The cost of dementia care around the world was estimated to be $600 billion in 2010. Most costs were not related to medical expenses, but the expense of social and informal caregiving.[4]

Worldwide, women live longer than men, thus women are more likely to be affected by dementia. This is especially significant as women age, because the rate of dementia doubles every 5 years after the age of 65. In many parts of the world, including Europe, Latin America, Australia, and areas outside of the Pacific region of Asia, female gender independently predicted a higher prevalence of dementia by approximately 20%.[1] This same finding was not found by the investigators in North America or the Pacific region of Asia. In addition, women outnumber men, with 55% of adults older than 60 being women in 2007.[5] The disproportionate numbers of women as compared with men continue to increase with age, especially in those older than 80, which is the age in which women are more likely to be affected by dementia.[5] In addition, women outnumber men in both developed and undeveloped countries, so dementia in women is not an isolated problem to the developed world.[5]

Studies have shown that two-thirds of Americans suffering from dementia are women.[6] Incidence studies are less clear, but do appear to show an increased incidence of dementia in women in the oldest old.[5] Similarly, it has been noted that Alzheimer dementia disproportionately affects women in both prevalence and severity. Some studies have shown that at a similar stage of Alzheimer dementia, women have more pronounced cognitive deficits than men[7]; however, the underlying mechanisms for these differences are unknown.[8]

There is also some evidence that women live longer than men after the development of dementia. Helmer and colleagues[9] found that regardless of the age of onset of Alzheimer dementia, survival was greater in women as compared with men. Although the investigators did not offer a theory about this phenomenon, they did note that this same finding has been demonstrated in other studies. The effect for longer survival in women showed a trend toward decreasing with advancing age.

Interestingly, women may be more concerned than men are about developing dementia and the potential consequences of developing aspects of this disease. Specifically, women were noted to have more fears about loss of independence, inability to help family members with their care needs, and forgetting important information, such as the identity of family members.[10]

There are many types of dementia that although sharing deficits in memory, cognition, and function, have very different etiologies and life course. Much of the research in the different dementias has not examined or reported on differences between genders or specifically studying women. The following assumes some knowledge of dementia disorders and is not meant to be an overview of the disorders, but rather a focus on what is known of gender differences in these disorders.

Alzheimer Disease

Alzheimer disease or Alzheimer dementia has a greater incidence and is more prevalent in women as compared with men.[11] This is especially true for the oldest old, with rates increasing disproportionately among the sexes at older ages.[12] In one study, the cumulative risk that someone would have dementia at the age of 95, if he or she lived that long, was calculated. The cumulative risk for a woman at the age of 65 to develop Alzheimer dementia at the age of 95 was found to be 0.22 as compared with 0.09 for men.[13] There are also differences in the clinical course of Alzheimer disease by gender. Men have been shown to have a higher mortality rate and a greater number of comorbidities than women. Women have been found to have a greater survival rate but with more disability.[14]

There has been much research as to the underlying genetics of Alzheimer disease and the illness is heterogeneous. APOE4, APP (amyloid precursor protein: chromosome 21), PSEN1 (presenilin 1: chromosome 14), and PSEN2 (presenilin 2: chromosome 1) are all genes implicated in the causality of Alzheimer dementia.[15] Of these genes, APOE4 is the greatest genetic risk factor, increasing one's lifetime risk to develop Alzheimer disease from 11% in men and 14% in women to 23% to 30% for APOE4 heterozygotes and 50% to 60% for APOE4 homozygotes. Female carriers of this gene (either heterozygotes or homozygotes) have a 7% to 10% greater lifetime risk than men with the same genotype.[16,17]

Behavioral aspects of Alzheimer disease

Almost all patients with Alzheimer dementia will develop behavioral symptoms during the course of the illness. Such symptoms are as much a part of the illness as the memory and cognitive features. These have been described as the neuropsychiatric symptoms of Alzheimer disease[15] and are shown in **Table 1**.

Depression is an independent risk factor for dementia with differences by gender. A prospective 14-year study of 1357 community-dwelling individuals in the Baltimore Longitudinal Study of Aging revealed that depressive symptoms significantly increased the risk of dementia in both men and women, but men particularly had an association to Alzheimer disease as compared with women.[18] Another large research project, the Women's Health Initiative Memory Study, examined 6376 women ages 65 to 79 and followed them for approximately 5 years. This study revealed that depressive symptoms at baseline were associated with significant increased risk for mild cognitive impairment (MCI) and probable dementia.[19]

Depressive symptoms have been described as more common in those with MCI or in the mild stage of dementia than later stages; however, depression is typically more difficult to diagnose and detect in more advanced stages, leading to missed depression diagnoses. In those stages, depression may present as agitation or aggression, decreased function and participation, and decreased appetite. Unfortunately, many of those symptoms are mistakenly attributed to the dementia process itself. The depression is thus missed and mistreated with sedatives or antipsychotics rather than antidepressants. Thus, many women with dementia and depression are not treated appropriately for their mood symptoms. Those with more neuropsychiatric symptoms and greater severity of symptoms have been found to have more functional limitations and caregiver burden, and are associated with a greater risk of nursing home placement.[20,21]

Among such symptoms, sexually inappropriate behaviors requiring treatment are seen more commonly in men than women with dementia. Although one study showed a similar prevalence of sexual behaviors in both men and women in dementia (8% vs

Table 1
Neuropsychiatric symptoms of Alzheimer disease

Symptom	Type
Affective symptoms	Depression, anxiety, apathy
Psychosis	Hallucinations (primarily visual and auditory), delusions
Disturbances of basic drives	Feeding, sleep, sexuality
Socially inappropriate behaviors	Disinhibition, hitting, yelling, aggression

7%), these were not sexual behaviors that reached the level of requiring treatment.[22] Although men are often successfully treated with an anti-androgen medication, such as medroxyprogesterone, for such behaviors, this approach is not successful with women. The authors' experience is that sexually inappropriate behaviors in women are typically disinhibited and may resemble maniclike sexual behaviors. Treatment with divalproex or buspirone has been successful in individual cases that are severe enough to warrant medication, when redirection or environmental adjustments prove unsuccessful.

Cognitive impairment

Research suggests that women with Alzheimer dementia may have more pronounced cognitive deficits than men. Laws and colleagues[11] recently performed a meta-analysis and found that men with Alzheimer dementia outperform women across multiple cognitive domains, with cognitive deficits in women being more pronounced in severity and number of domains affected. There is also evidence that women may deteriorate faster than men cognitively in the early stages of Alzheimer dementia. Theories for this include age-related estrogen loss in women or a greater cognitive reserve in men.[11] Risk factors for progression of disease also may be present more in women, including more severe periventricular white matter abnormalities on neuroimaging, and poorer global cognitive functioning. Older age, worse depressive symptoms, and being positive for APOE4 were risk factors for more rapid progression in women.[23]

Neuroimaging offers some clues as to why women have a worse disease course than men with Alzheimer dementia. Neuroimaging is an important part of the workup of a patient with suspected Alzheimer dementia in the form of providing supporting diagnostic evidence, and ruling out alternative causes of cognitive decline. Medial temporal and hippocampal atrophy can provide supportive diagnostic information.[17,24] Recent research has found that hippocampal volumetric integrity decreased more rapidly in women with Alzheimer disease as compared with men.[25,26]

The treatment for Alzheimer dementia involves both behavioral and psychosocial interventions as well as pharmacologic management. The importance of a dependable caregiver cannot be overstated and unfortunately it may be more difficult for women with dementia to have access to adequate caregivers, as their spouse may already be deceased or unwilling or unable to serve as a caregiver. Caregivers should be educated on the patient's disease course; specific areas of need, safety, and available resources; and resources for caregiver burnout.[17]

Concerning pharmacologic management, the acetylcholinesterase inhibitors are the treatment recommended for the initial phases of the disease. These include donepezil, galantamine, and rivastigmine. For later stages of the disease course (moderate to severe), the N-methyl-D-aspartate antagonist memantine is used.[17] There is some evidence that women respond better to acetylcholinesterase inhibitors than men. Scacchi and colleagues[27] conducted a study with 184 patients with Alzheimer dementia taking rivastigmine and donepezil who were followed over a 15-month period. They found that women appeared to be more sensitive to the effects of acetylcholinesterase inhibitors than men and postulated that sex variants of the estrogen receptor, alpha ESR 1 may be a contributing factor.[26,27]

Lewy Body Dementias

Lewy body dementias include Parkinson disease dementia (PDD) and dementia with Lewy bodies (DLB). DLB is a common degenerative dementia; however, with much clinical overlap of symptoms with Alzheimer disease. It is characterized by fluctuating cognition (need to rule out delirium), recurrent and prominent visual hallucinations that are well formed and detailed, rapid eye movement sleep behaviors, and features of parkinsonism. Diagnosis is clinical and presumptive and can be definitely diagnosed only at autopsy, with the finding of Lewy bodies in the cortical brain regions. PDD is diagnosed in patients who have had a diagnosis of Parkinson disease for at least a year, but usually many years, and then develop cognitive symptoms, which occurs in approximately 30% to 40% of patients. Research has shown that women are at less risk to develop PDD than men. With PDD, the incidence is similar for men and women except for the oldest age group that is mostly represented by men.[15,28,29] Similarly, women are found to have a lower incidence of Lewy body dementia than men at all ages. Thus, Lewy body dementias overall appear to disproportionately affect men. As far as is currently known, there do not appear to be differences in symptoms or course of these dementias between genders.

Vascular Dementia

Vascular dementia is due to vascular insults to the central nervous system. It is one of the most common causes of dementia following Alzheimer dementia. As with Alzheimer dementia, the risk of vascular dementia increases with advancing age, but the rate of increase is not as great as with Alzheimer dementia.[30,31] There appear to be no differences in the prevalence of vascular dementia between men and women.[13]

With regard to the effect of this disease on women, research suggests that prestroke dementia is more common in women than poststroke dementia.[30,32] Thus, a greater proportion of women in the study already had dementia at the time of their stroke.

CARING FOR WOMEN WITH DEMENTIA

Research has shown the importance of maintenance of identity for patients with dementia, and the ways caretakers may help maintain this. For example, in many cultures, women serve as caretakers for their family. However, women who are afflicted with dementia begin to lose the ability to care for themselves and others. This may lead to a role reversal in which they receive care from family members for whom they have cared for in the past. Ways to reconnect to behaviors and activities connected with their identity before the dementia can be very important to patients. As an example, researchers have described the use of handbags in female patients with dementia as a source of identity along with the objects that they contain.[33] Handbags were also found to be useful reminders of identity when moving from their familiar home to an assisted living facility. Families and caregivers are encouraged to think about the role of the woman with dementia and enhance the role identity, whatever it may be. Dr. Holroyd, recalls a patient who had been a surgeon who was given a clipboard so she could “go on rounds” walking up and down the hallway of the nursing home. Similarly, many women with dementia enjoy holding baby dolls and seem very comforted by identification as prior roles as mothers. Maintenance of identity is also important to the families and spouses of those women afflicted with dementia, who often work to help their spouses keep a normal gendered appearance.[2]

Patients may enjoy activities, such as having their nails done, doing washing or cooking activities, planting gardens, or interacting with children or pets, as a connection to prior roles and identities. Those with dementia want to feel useful and may enjoy helping with activities more than being entertained or watching TV or a movie. A patient of Dr. Holroyd who had 10 children was frequently agitated until she was given piles of clothes to fold, which she would do for hours and was very comforting to her, connecting her to her past identity and life.

In addition, the decreasing independence that occurs in dementia can be a very difficult adjustment. This loss of independence often leads to conflict between the person suffering from dementia and their caregivers, as the sufferer tries to maintain their independence. This usually begins with inability to perform independent activities of daily living (iADLs), for example paying bills or managing a checkbook.[34] Ward-Griffin and colleagues[35] discussed the phenomenon of "grateful guilt" when mothers are forced to rely on their daughters for care assistance. The investigators found the idea of "retiring" from an activity to be a more positive and palatable way to view giving up such an activity rather than being told they can no longer do it. In such an interaction, it may be pointed out, for example, that the woman's husband has retired from his job, but she is still doing her jobs at home (eg, doing the checkbook, cooking) and now it is her turn to "retire" from such activities. This allows her to "deserve" to retire from the activity rather than feeling shamed or humiliated that she can no longer do it.

Medically, health issues may dramatically worsen cognition or behaviors in dementia. Urinary tract infections (UTIs) are one of the most common causes of behavioral disturbance in female patients with dementia. UTI's may present with behavioral issues rather than symptoms such as urinary frequency, burning, pain, or fever. New-onset psychosis in a patient with dementia must always rule out UTI. Women's bladders lose function with age and become less likely to fully empty, thus increasing the chance of UTI, as well as requiring longer courses of antibiotic treatment to fully eradicate the infection. All patients should have follow-up urine cultures several days after their last day of antibiotic treatment to ensure the UTI is gone. At times, recurrent UTIs may require prophylactic antibiotics to prevent further infections, although this may cause issues with bacterial resistance or vulnerability to *Clostridium difficile*. A useful alternative is prescribing over-the-counter cranberry pills 3 times a day with meals to acidify the urine, making it a more hostile environment for the bacteria to infect. As with UTIs, any infection or systemic medical illness can dramatically worsen cognition or behaviors so any change in such symptoms requires a close physical examination and appropriate laboratory tests so medical issues can be promptly addressed.

WOMEN AND CAREGIVING

Besides more frequently having dementia, women are also more often placed in the caregiving role to those with dementia. Studies have demonstrated that up to 60% to 70% of caregivers for patients with dementia are women.[2] Most of these women are the adult daughters or spouses of patients with dementia. Most of these caregiving women are older than 65, thus adding to the difficulty of the caregiving burden. In addition, women are also more likely to spend increased amounts of time in caregiving activities than men.[36] The reasons for this are likely multifactorial, but one theory is that women are less likely to work outside of the home.[36,37] Another theory is that women end up being caregivers more frequently because of cultural expectations of women. Family expectations may be that daughters or wives will provide caregiving for such patients. Many women may not even consider themselves caregivers when asked, as they see that as their normal role within the family.

Because of their increased time spent in caregiving activities, women also have tended to have more interference in their work and social relationships when compared with male caregivers.[36] Studies have demonstrated conflicting results as to whether women experience greater joy than men from caregiving.[36] When evaluating caregiver burden between the sexes, Sharma and colleagues[36] found in their literature review that some, but not all studies suggest greater caregiver burden in women.

For any caregiver, the transition to the caregiving role may be difficult, as this leads to a change in the identity of the relationship with those who receive the care. For example, women may change from the typical roles of daughter and/or wife to caregiver.[2] Finally, the women who serve as caregivers often must learn new skills to assume this role. In most relationships, persons may carry out or be responsible for different roles and tasks in that relationship. Women caregivers not only have to care for their loved one with dementia, but also may have to assume unfamiliar tasks that were previously handled by the person with dementia in their lives. This can add additional stress and burden for the women involved.[2]

SUMMARY

Despite the progress made in the understanding of the etiology, neuropathophysiology, and treatment of different types of dementia, such disorders continue to pose significant and increasing health problems worldwide. Although it is clear that certain dementias are more common or severe in women, little research has been done in understanding the basis for these gender differences, which would be important in understanding the etiology of dementia in general. Further research is obviously needed not only for all dementia disorders, but specifically to further understand the basis for dementia in women.

REFERENCES

1. Price M, Renata M, Emiliano A, et al. The global prevalence of dementia: a systematic review and metaanalysis. Alzheimers Dement 2013;9(1):63–75.
2. Erol R, Brooker D, Peel E. Alzheimer's Disease International. Women and dementia: a global research review. 2015. Available at: https://www.alz.co.uk/sites/default/files/pdfs/Women-and-Dementia.pdf. Accessed May 5, 2016.
3. Alzheimer's Disease International. The global impact of dementia 2013-2050. 2013. Available at: https://www.alz.co.uk/research/GlobalImpactDementia2013.pdf. Accessed May 5, 2016.
4. Wortmann M. Dementia: a global health priority—highlights from an ADI and World Health Organization report. Alzheimers Res Ther 2012;4(5):40.
5. Braun J. Dementia: a woman's global health issue. Washington, DC: Alzheimer's Disease International; 2012.
6. Alzheimers Disease International. The global impact of dementia: prevalence, incidence, cost, and trends. London: Alzheimer's Disease International; 2015. Available at: https://www.alz.co.uk/research/WorldAlzheimerReport2015.pdf. Accessed May 5, 2016.
7. Irvine K, Laws KR, Gale TM, et al. Greater cognitive deterioration in women than men with Alzheimer's disease: a meta analysis. J Clin Exp Neuropsychol 2012;34(9):989–98.
8. Carter CL, Resnick EM, Mallampalli M, et al. Sex and gender differences in Alzheimer's disease: recommendations for future research. J Womens Health 2012;21(10):1018–23.
9. Helmer C, Jolly P, Letenneur L, et al. Mortality with dementia: results from a French prospective community-based cohort. Am J Epidemiol 2001;154(7):642–8.
10. Alzheimer's Association. Alzheimer's disease facts and figures. Alzheimers Dement 2014;10(2):e47–92. Available at: https://www.alz.org/downloads/facts_figures_2014.pdf. Accessed May 5, 2016.

11. Laws KR, Irvine K, Gale TM. Sex differences in cognitive impairment in Alzheimer's disease. World J Psychiatry 2016;6(1):54–65.
12. Lobo A, Launer LJ, Fratiglioni L, et al. Prevalence of dementia and major subtypes in Europe: a collaborative study of population-based cohorts. Neurologic diseases in the elderly research group. Neurology 2000;54:S4–9.
13. Andersen K, Launer LJ, Dewey ME, et al. Gender differences in the incidence of AD and vascular dementia: The EURODEM Studies. EURODEM Incidence Research Group. Neurology 1999;53:1992–7.
14. Sinforiani E, Citterio A, Zucchella C, et al. Impact of gender differences on the outcome of Alzheimer's disease. Dement Geriatr Cogn Disord 2010;30:147–54.
15. Lyketsos C. Dementia and milder cognitive syndromes. In: Blazer DG, Steffens DC, editors. Essentials of geriatric psychiatry. Second edition. Arlington (VA): American Psychiatric Publishing; 2012. p. 107–24.
16. Genin E, Hannequin D, Wallon D, et al. *APOE* and Alzheimer disease: a major gene with semi-dominant inheritance. Mol Psychiatry 2011;16(9):903–7.
17. Schletens P, Blennow K, Breteler M, et al. Alzheimer's disease. Lancet 2016; 388(10043):505–17.
18. Dal Forno G, Palermo MT, Donohue JE, et al. Depressive symptoms, sex and risk for Alzheimer's disease. Ann Neurol 2005;57:381–7.
19. Goveas JS, Espeland MA, Woods NF, et al. Depressive symptoms and incidence of mild cognitive impairment and probably dementia in elderly women: the women's Health Initiative Memory Study. J Am Geriatr Soc 2011;59:57–66.
20. Okura T, Plassman BL, Steffens DC, et al. Prevalence of neuropsychiatric symptoms and their association with functional limitations in older adults in the United States: the aging, demographics, and memory study. J Am Geriatr Soc 2010; 58(2):330–7.
21. Bergvall N, Brinck P, Eek D, et al. Relative importance of patient disease indicators on informal care and caregiver burden in Alzheimer's disease. Int Psychogeriatr 2011;23:73–85.
22. Burns A, Jacoby R, Levy R. Psychiatric phenomena in Alzheimer's disease IV. Disorders of behavior. Br J Psychiatry 1990;157:86–94.
23. Kim S, Kim MJ, Kim S, et al. Gender differences in risk factors for transition from mild cognitive impairment to Alzheimer's disease: a CREDOS study. Compr Psychiatry 2015;62:114–22.
24. Frisoni GB, Fox NC, Jack CR, et al. The clinical use of structural MRI in Alzheimer disease. Nat Rev Neurol 2010;6(2):67–77.
25. Ardekani B, Convit A, Bachman AH. Analysis of the MIRIAS data shows sex differences in hippocampal atrophy progression. J Alzheimers Dis 2016;50:3.
26. Mazure CM, Swendsen J. Sex differences in Alzheimer's disease and other dementias. Lancet Neurol 2016;15(5):451–2.
27. Scacchi R, Gambina G, Broggio E, et al. Sex and *ESR1* genotype may influence the response to treatment with donepezil and rivastigmine in patients with Alzheimer's disease. Int J Geriatr Psychiatry 2014;29:610–5.
28. Hughes TA, Ross HF, Musa S, et al. A 10-year study of the incidence of and factors predicting dementia in Parkinson's disease. Neurology 2000;54:1596–602.
29. McKeith I, Dickson DW, Lowe J, et al. Diagnosis and management of dementia with Lewy bodies: third report of the DLB consortium. Neurology 2005;65(12): 1863–72.
30. O'Brien JT, Thomas A. Vascular dementia. Lancet 2015;386(10004):1698–7106.
31. Jorm AF, Jolley D. The incidence of dementia: a meta-analysis. Neurology 1998; 51:728–33.

32. Pendlebury S, Rothwell P. Prevalence, incidence, and factors associated with pre-stroke and post-stroke dementia: a systematic review and meta-analysis. Lancet Neurol 2009;8:1006–18.
33. Buse C, Twigg J. Women with dementia and their handbags: negotiating identity, privacy and 'home' through material culture. J Aging Stud 2014;30:14–22.
34. Borley G, Sixsmith J, Church S. How does a woman with Alzheimer's disease make sense of becoming cared for? Dementia (Lond) 2014;15(6):1405–21.
35. Ward-Griffin C, Bol N, Oudshoorn A. Perspectives of women with dementia receiving care from their adult daughters. Can J Nurs Res 2006;38(1):120–46.
36. Sharma N, Chakrabarti S, Grover S. Gender differences in caregiving among family—caregivers of people with mental illnesses. World J Psychiatry 2016; 6(1):7–17.
37. Almada A. Gender and caregiving: a study among Hispanic and non-Hispanic white frail elders [Master's Thesis]. Blacksburg (VA): Virginia Polytechnic Institute and State University; 2001. Available at: http://www.scholar.lib.vt.edu. Accessed June 10, 2016.

Mental Health in Sexual Minority and Transgender Women

Julie K. Schulman, MD[a,*], Laura Erickson-Schroth, MD, MA[b]

KEYWORDS

- Lesbian • Bisexual • Transgender • Sexual minority • Mental health
- Minority stress

KEY POINTS

- Sexual minority and transgender women experience increased rates of societal discrimination, harassment, and violence. Minority stress theory links these experiences to increased rates of mental illness and substance use disorders in those groups.
- For many mental health conditions and substance use disorders, bisexual women are at even higher risk than are lesbians. This is partly attributable to stigmatization of bisexual women in both heterosexual and gay communities.
- Family acceptance, social support, and community connectedness have been shown to contribute to resilience in sexual minority and transgender women. Sexual minority and transgender women often avoid mental health and substance abuse treatment because of past or feared negative experiences with clinicians or treatment programs.
- Clinicians should not rely on their sexual minority and transgender clients to educate them. Instead, they should seek out education from other sources in order to develop cultural competence in working with such clients.

INTRODUCTION

Terminology related to sexuality and gender identity is constantly evolving. Most clinicians are familiar with the acronym LGBT, which refers to the lesbian, gay, bisexual,

This article originally appeared in the *Psychiatric Clinics of North America*, Volume 40, Issue 2, June 2017.
Disclosure Statement: The authors have nothing to disclose.
[a] Department of Psychiatry, Allen Hospital, 5141 Broadway, 3 River East, New York, NY 10034, USA; [b] Department of Psychiatry, Mount Sinai Beth Israel, 10 Nathan D. Perlman Place, New York, NY 10003, USA
* Corresponding author.
E-mail address: js1781@cumc.columbia.edu

Med Clin N Am 103 (2019) 723–733
http://dx.doi.org/10.1016/j.mcna.2019.02.005 medical.theclinics.com

and transgender community.* The first 3 terms, lesbian, gay, and bisexual, are used to define one's *sexual orientation*, which refers to the gender of those to whom a person is attracted, and with whom they may have sexual or romantic relationships. Transgender is a term that defines one's *gender identity*, which is a person's sense of their own gender. A person whose gender identity matches the gender they were assigned at birth is *cisgender*, whereas a person whose gender identity does not match the gender they were assigned at birth is *transgender*. Although LGB and transgender people share certain life experiences, particularly with regard to stigmatization and discrimination, the 2 communities are also quite distinct in many ways.

The term *sexual minority women (SMW)* is used in this article to refer to all women who may be defined as nonheterosexual. There are 3 generally accepted dimensions of sexual orientation: sexual identity (the term someone uses to describe herself, such as lesbian, bisexual, or queer), sexual attraction, and sexual behavior. SMW includes women who would be considered nonheterosexual in at least 1 of these 3 dimensions. Consequently, SMW includes those who self-identify as lesbian or bisexual; those who identify as heterosexual but report having sexual attraction to women; and those who identify as heterosexual but report having had female sexual partners. In discussing specific research, the authors endeavor to use the most specific term possible to refer to the subpopulation that was studied. Unless otherwise specified, when the term lesbian, bisexual, or gay is used, it refers to people who self-identify as such.

Although there are gender minority women who are not transgender, for example, women who identify as genderfluid, bigender, or genderqueer, this article focuses only on transgender women. *Transgender women* are individuals who were assigned a male gender at birth but identify as female. Transgender women are a diverse group and may or may not wish to take hormones or have any type of surgery. Transgender women are often assumed to be heterosexual (or *androphilic*, attracted to men), but many identify as lesbian, bisexual, or queer, or are sexually attracted to or sexually active with women (*gynephilic*). In fact, in the National Transgender Discrimination Survey, only 23% of transgender women identified as heterosexual.[1] Unfortunately, most studies of mixed-gender populations, even when they allow subjects to identify themselves as transgender, do not ask further questions to allow data separation of transgender women from transgender men. In this article, if no gender specifier is used after the word transgender in discussing a research finding, it means the subjects were a mixed-gender group.

TRAUMA AND MINORITY STRESS

Minority stress is a term initially used by Brooks[2] in her work with lesbian women. She defined it as "a state intervening between the sequential antecedent stressors of culturally sanctioned, categorically ascribed inferior status, resultant prejudice and discrimination, the impact of these forces on the cognitive structure of the individual, and consequent readjustment or adaptational failure." Meyer[3] adopted a

* In some cases, the letter Q is added to LGBT, to include the term "queer." Queer is a word which may be used to describe anyone identifying as non-heterosexual or non-cisgender. This would include anyone who is LGBT, but also multiple other categories, eg, those who are asexual, are uncertain of their sexual orientation, or do not identify with any gender. However, this term is one that was initially neutral but was then used only in a derogatory manner for many years, and it still carries a highly negative implication when used by someone who opposes equal treatment of people with non-heterosexual or non-cisgender identities. Therefore, some people are offended by the term, and you should never use it to refer to someone directly unless they have already indicated that they do not mind if you do so.

similar conceptualization for his *minority stress theory*, in which he connected not only the discrimination and violence that LGB individuals face but also the "juxtaposition of minority and dominant values and the resultant conflict with the social environment" with increased rates of mental health disparities. The minority stress model has since been expanded to other populations, including transgender people.[4]

Meyer's model, as he outlined it in 2003, proposes 3 ways in which sexual and gender minorities are subjected to minority stress.[5] The first is via the external events that occur in an LGBT person's life, such as harassment or discrimination, which Meyer called *distal stressors*. The other 2 are *proximal stressors*, which are personal and subjective. The first is the anticipation of such events, leading to increased vigilance or concealment of one's identity, and the second is the internalization of external negative beliefs and societal prejudice, which is referred to as *internalized homophobia* (or *internalized transphobia*.) Minority stress is chronic, and it is experienced as an additional burden, above and beyond that caused by the life stressors that all people face.

It has been very well documented that transgender people face increased rates of discrimination and violence, and that transgender women are at especially high risk. In the largest community-based study to date, the National Transgender Discrimination Survey, conducted in 2008 with 6450 respondents from all 50 states, DC, Puerto Rico, Guam, and the US Virgin Islands, 47% of respondents reported being denied promotion, fired, or not hired because of their gender identity.[1] Nineteen percent reported being refused a home or apartment because they were transgender, and 55% of those attempting to access the shelter system experienced harassment by shelter staff or residents. Discrimination extends to the health care system: 19% of respondents had been refused health care due to their gender identity, and 28% had postponed medical care because of discrimination. Societal stigma and discrimination can also have directly fatal consequences. In a report from the National Coalition of Anti-Violence Programs, in 2013, 72% of all reported LGBTQ or human immunodeficiency virus–related hate violence fatalities were transgender women, of whom all but one was a woman of color.[6]

SMW also face significant minority stress, and as surveys have become more exact in defining sexual orientation, it has become apparent that women who identify as bisexual are at higher risk than their lesbian counterparts for many mental health and substance use disorders. At least some of this risk is likely attributable to the stigmatization that bisexual women experience in both gay and heterosexual communities, where they may be stereotyped as either lesbians in denial, or heterosexual women who are just experimenting. Bisexual women also have the highest risk of having experienced sexual assaults or domestic violence. In the 2010 Centers for Disease Control and Prevention report on Intimate Partner and Sexual Violence, bisexual women had a higher lifetime prevalence of rape by any perpetrator (46.1%) than lesbians (13.1%) or heterosexual women (17.4%) as well as other types of sexual assault (74.9% vs 46.4% and 43.3%, respectively).[7] In addition, 61.1% of bisexual women report a history of rape, physical violence, or stalking in a relationship, compared with 43.8% of lesbians (of whom two-thirds reported only female perpetrators) and 35% of heterosexual women.

More recently, researchers have begun to explore not only those experiences that may lead to poor mental health outcomes in LGBT people but also factors that may contribute to positive coping in the face of adversity. Family acceptance of LGBT adolescents predicts greater self-esteem and general health, and also protects against depression, substance abuse, and suicidal ideation and behaviors.[8] Peer and general social support as well as community connectedness has also been shown to contribute to resilience in LGBT populations.[9–11] Studies have been inconclusive regarding whether "outness" (ie, openness about one's minority sexual or gender identity) is protective for LGBT individuals, and it is likely this is more nuanced. Being out eliminates the proximal stressor of concealing one's identity, but in some situations, the increased exposure to discrimination and prejudice by other people may outweigh this benefit.

MENTAL HEALTH DISPARITIES

Body Image and Eating Disorders

Although lesbians are more likely to be overweight or obese than heterosexual women,[12] studies suggest that they are less likely than heterosexual women of the same body mass index to have body dissatisfaction.[13–15] It is less clear how nonlesbian SMW fare with regard to body image in comparison to heterosexual or lesbian women.

Unfortunately, there are little data on the prevalence of disordered eating or eating disorders in adult SMW. Koh and Ross[16] surveyed women from 33 health care sites across the US, a convenience sample weighted toward SMW but with a heterosexual control group, and found that self-identified bisexual women were approximately twice as likely to have a history of an eating disorder as heterosexual women, while lesbians were only slightly more likely than heterosexual women to have had an eating disorder. A recent national survey of college students found that among cisgender female students, SMW were significantly less likely than heterosexual women to have taken diet pills or vomited/used laxatives in the past month, while no significant distinction could be made in the rates of past-year diagnosis of anorexia or bulimia, likely due to the low prevalence of these disorders.[17]

Although some transgender women struggle with body dysphoria, especially before physically transitioning, there is little formal research in this area and virtually none with regard to eating disorders. Most has been done with community-based samples, such as one which found that transgender women at various stages of transition, who had no significant difference in BMI from cisgender female subjects, were more dissatisfied than cisgender women on scales of weight concern, shape concern, and body dissatisfaction.[18] With regard to eating disorders, there have been two large studies that have provided data on mixed-gender transgender subjects in comparison to cisgender subjects.[17,19] However, neither study allows for a direct comparison of the rate of eating disorders in transgender women with that of cisgender women, so the utility of these studies is limited.

Mood and Anxiety

Even though most SMW, like heterosexual women, have no mental health issues, adult SMW as a whole have higher rates of mood and anxiety disorders than do heterosexual women. Several large population-based studies and meta-analyses have confirmed these findings for a variety of mood and anxiety disorders.[20–23]

However, the overall numbers obscure important differences in the various subtypes of SMW. There is increasing evidence that bisexual women, particularly those who are self-identified but also those defined by sexual attraction or behavior, are at higher risk for mental health issues than women who are exclusively homosexual in orientation. Self-identified or behaviorally-identified bisexual women have never been found to have lower rates of any mood or anxiety disorders or psychiatric symptoms in comparison to heterosexuals in any national study, and have rarely been found to have any of these at a rate equal to that of heterosexuals. On the other hand, in an increasing number of nationwide population studies, self-identified or behaviorally-identified lesbian women have either the same or even lower rates of some mood or anxiety disorders or psychiatric symptoms in comparison to heterosexual women.

For example, in a 2004 to 2005 national population survey, self-identified bisexual women had the highest risk of lifetime or past- year mood or anxiety disorders, followed by self-identified lesbians and heterosexual women. Women with a history of only same-sex behavior were at even lower risk than heterosexual women for lifetime mood disorders and trended toward lower risk than heterosexual women for lifetime anxiety disorder and for past-year mood or anxiety disorders.[20] A recent article by Gonzales and colleagues,[24] using data from the National Health Interview Survey of 2013 to 2014, found that in comparison to heterosexual women, bisexual women had significantly higher rates of moderate or severe psychological distress, with odds ratios of 2.17 and 3.69, respectively. Lesbian women were only significantly higher than heterosexual women for moderate distress, with a more modest odds ratio of 1.34.

If minority stress theory is correct, we would expect the rates of psychiatric disorders or symptoms in lesbians to gradually approach or even equal those of heterosexual women, as long as the heterosexual community continues to become more accepting of lesbians. Similarly, we would expect this to happen with bisexual and transgender women. However, this will be a longer process for bisexual and transgender women. For bisexual women, attitudes will have to change in both the lesbian and heterosexual communities, and for transgender women, it will have to change in both the male and female cisgender communities. In addition, it typically takes longer for society to accept people with minority identities as equals when doing so necessitates changing a concept traditionally viewed as binary (eg, gay/straight, or male/female) to one that is non-binary.

Numerous studies have shown increased rates of depression in transgender populations.[25–27] In a study of 191 transgender women in Ontario, depression was estimated at 61%.[28] Anxiety in transgender women is less well studied and is typically not the primary endpoint when it is included in research. In a 2013 study of coping mechanisms in transgender individuals, 40% of transgender women had anxiety symptoms.[29]

Suicidality and Self-Harm

Studies have consistently found higher rates of reported suicidality and suicide attempts in SMW compared with heterosexual women. However, the magnitude of the risk has been hard to quantify. A recent review and meta-analysis of studies found that an average of 20% of LGB adults reported a history of suicide attempts in community-based surveys, whereas only 11% reported this in population-based surveys, compared with 4% for heterosexuals in population-based surveys; they did not report gender-specific data.[30]

A meta-analysis of studies in adults published in 2008 found that SMW had a relative risk of 2.31 for past-year suicidal ideation and 1.55 for lifetime suicidal ideation in comparison to heterosexual women; the relative risks for suicide attempt were 2.45 for past year and 1.82 for lifetime.[21] However, small sample sizes and selection bias limited the quality of the studies available. Blosnich and colleagues[31] used population-based data from the California Quality of Life Surveys and found that in comparison to heterosexual women, lifetime suicidal ideation risk was elevated 3-fold in bisexual women, and

2-fold in lesbians and mostly heterosexual women (those with a heterosexual identity but with a history of same-sex partner in adulthood). Bisexual women also had a near 6-fold adjusted relative risk of lifetime suicide attempts, whereas lesbians and mostly heterosexual women were at less than 3-fold greater risk.

No one knows whether SMW have a higher mortality rate from suicide than heterosexual women, because sexual orientation data are not collected on death certificates, and the mortality rate is dependent on both the frequency of attempts and the potential lethality of the methods used. One recent study suggested that there may be a 6-fold higher rate of completed suicides in women who have ever had a same-sex partner compared with those who have not. However, it was based on a data set that used probabilistic matching to link participants in a national survey with mortality data from the National Death Index and should be interpreted with caution.[32,33]

Suicidality and self-harm are also major concerns in transgender populations. Varying definitions of suicidal ideation and suicide attempts make exact estimates of suicidality difficult, but studies have found that 25% to 76% of transgender people consider or attempt suicide.[34] In the National Transgender Discrimination Survey, 41% of respondents reported having attempted suicide.[1] Just as for SMW, however, we do not know the rate of completed suicides. Nonsuicidal self-harm among transgender people is less well characterized, but there is evidence to suggest that cutting and other self-harming behaviors are more common in transgender people, and especially trans youth.[35,36] Of note, there is a common misperception that transgender people's self-harming behaviors are genitally focused, but genital mutilation in transgender people, like in cisgender people, is rare, with only a few published case reports.

SUBSTANCE ABUSE

Several large population-based studies suggest that SMW are at higher risk of cigarette smoking[24,37,38] and problematic alcohol use or alcohol use disorder[24,39,40] than are heterosexual women. SMW are also more likely to have used drugs or to have substance use disorders.[40,41] Although some of this is attributable to minority stress, there are other contributory factors, such as social learning. In the United States, gay bars have played a vital role as gathering spaces for LGBT individuals for well over a century, and in 1969, a police raid on a gay bar in New York City called the Stonewall Inn became a pivotal moment in the contemporary gay civil rights movement when the patrons and community members fought back. Although gay bars no longer play such a central role in LGBT communities, many older LGBT adults nonetheless remember their first trip to a gay bar, often requiring fake identification to enter while still below the legal drinking age, as an important rite of passage in "coming out." Not surprisingly, at least one study has confirmed that SMW endorse more tolerant social norms for alcohol and drug use.[42]

Transgender people also report higher rates of alcohol and drug abuse than their cisgender counterparts.[1,43,44] Certain drugs such as methamphetamine and amyl nitrate, which are relatively more common choices as drugs of abuse in some urban gay communities than they are in similarly located heterosexual ones, may also be relatively more common in similarly located transgender communities.[45] Substance use in transgender communities is complicated by many different factors. For example, transgender women engaging in sex work may abuse substances to facilitate their work, or conversely, may be more likely to engage in sex work if already abusing substances.[46]

TREATMENT CONSIDERATIONS

Barriers to Care

Sexual minority and transgender women face several barriers in accessing quality care. In a survey by Lambda Legal, 28.5% of sexual minority respondents and 73% of transgender respondents reported concerns that medical personnel would treat them differently. In the same survey, 9.1% of sexual minority respondents and 59.1% of transgender respondents said they feared they would be refused medical service.[47] Even if they are willing to seek help, sexual minority and transgender people often find that their providers are not well educated about their needs. A 2011 study in the *Journal of the American Medical Association* revealed that medical schools, on average, teach only 5 hours of sexual minority and transgender–related content over the entire 4 years.[48]

Many LGBT people are especially wary of mental health providers because of a history of pathologization of homosexuality and transgender identity. Homosexuality was considered a mental illness by the American Psychiatric Association until 1973. Transgender-related diagnoses remain in the *Diagnostic and Statistical Manual of Mental Disorders* (DSM), currently as Gender Dysphoria in the DSM-5. Many think this new diagnosis is an improvement on the DSM-IV's Gender Identity Disorder, but others think that it leads to continued pathologization and should be removed. The main argument for continued inclusion in the DSM has been that if it were removed, many transgender people in the United States would lose access to hormone treatment or surgery, because insurers typically require a formal medical diagnosis. However, a proposal has been made to rename Gender Identity Disorder as Gender Incongruence in the next International Classification of Diseases (ICD-11), due in 2018, and move it out of the behavioral health section, thus reducing the stigma associated with the diagnosis.[49]

Pathologization is not the only reason that LGBT people distance themselves from mental health providers. For many years, it was standard to approach sexual and gender minority clients using reparative/conversion therapy, which attempted to change the sexual orientation or gender identity of the client. Despite evidence that this practice is ineffective and harmful, some practitioners continue to use it. Several states have begun to ban its use with minors.[50]

Transgender people have an especially fraught relationship with mental health providers. In addition to pathologization and attempts at reparative therapy, mental health providers often serve as "gatekeepers" for access to hormones or surgical procedures. In large cities, trans people can now typically access hormones directly through a process of informed consent with a primary care provider, but those who live in more rural areas may not have this option. When meeting with mental health providers, many trans people feel they have to provide life stories that align with traditional narratives of trans identity in order to receive letters for hormones or surgeries. This can create an atmosphere of mistrust and poor therapeutic alliance.

Providing Quality Care

There are several steps that individual clinicians and agencies can take to improve the quality of care provided to sexual minority and transgender women. From the moment a client steps through the door, the posters in the waiting room, the friendliness and LGBT awareness of the office staff, and the availability of gender-neutral restrooms signal the presence of a welcoming or hostile environment. Once in session, clients often pay close attention to the language a clinician uses, in addition to the clinician's willingness to admit areas of incomplete knowledge.

Psychiatrists can begin to improve their work with sexual and gender minority women by simply listening carefully before formulating ideas about them. A person's symptoms may be related to her gender or sexuality, or she may be struggling with an unrelated issue, in which case her sexuality or gender identity should become a routine part of the social and medical history and not take over the session. Psychiatrists should use their clients' language and respect their stated names and pronouns, both in session with the client and outside of session when talking with other staff members.

It is not enough, though, to learn from individual clients. Clinicians working with sexual minority and transgender women should seek out educational experiences by reading articles, using online educational resources for physicians or mental health clinicians, and attending conferences.

Finally, psychiatrists can be more than simply clinicians. Given our privilege as physicians, we can be advocates for our clients, helping to make meaningful change in their lives and the lives of other sexual minority and transgender women. There are many ways to be an advocate, including speaking up in workplaces or within organizations, writing about salient issues, reaching out to other clinicians on behalf of clients, calling ahead to let a primary care provider know that a patient is concerned about sensitivity during a certain examination, or writing a letter on behalf of a client for hormonal therapy or surgery.

REFERENCES

1. Grant JM, Mottet LA, Tanis J, et al. Injustice at every turn: a report of the national transgender discrimination survey. Washington, DC: National Center for Transgender Equality; 2011.
2. Brooks VR. The theory of minority stress. In: Brooks VR, editor. Minority stress and lesbian women. Lexington (MA): Lexington Books; 1981. p. 71–90.
3. Meyer IH. Minority stress and mental health in gay men. J Health Soc Behav 1995;36(1):38–56. Available at: http://www.jstor.org/stable/2137286.
4. Hendricks ML, Testa RJ. A conceptual framework for clinical work with transgender and gender nonconforming clients: an adaptation of the minority stress model. Prof Psychol Res Pract 2012;43(5):460–7.
5. Meyer IH. Prejudice, social stress, and mental health in lesbian, gay, and bisexual populations: conceptual issues and research evidence. Psychol Bull 2003; 129(5):674–97.
6. Ahmed O, Jindasurat C. Lesbian, Gay, Bisexual, Transgender, Queer and HIV-Affected Hate Violence in 2013. New York: National Coalition of Anti-Violence Programs; 2014. Available at: http://www.avp.org/storage/documents/2013_ncavp_hvreport_final.pdf. Accessed March 9, 2017.
7. Walters ML, Chen J, Breiding MJ. The national intimate partner and sexual violence survey: 2010 findings on victimization by sexual orientation. Natl Intim 2013;1–48. http://dx.doi.org/10.1037/e541522013-001.
8. Ryan C, Russell ST, Huebner D, et al. Family acceptance in adolescence and the health of LGBT young adults. J Child Adolesc Psychiatr Nurs 2010;23(4):205–13.
9. Bockting WO, Miner MH, Swinburne Romine RE, et al. Stigma, mental health, and resilience in an online sample of the US transgender population. Am J Public Health 2013;103(5):943–51.
10. Testa RJ, Jimenez CL, Rankin S. Risk and resilience during transgender identity development: the effects of awareness and engagement with other transgender people on affect. J Gay Lesbian Ment Health 2014;18(1):31–46.

11. Hatzenbuehler ML, Keyes KM, McLaughlin KA. The protective effects of social/contextual factors on psychiatric morbidity in LGB populations. Int J Epidemiol 2011;40(4):1071–80.
12. Gay and Lesbian Medical Association and LGBT health experts. Healthy People 2010 Companion Document for Lesbian, Gay, Bisexual, and Transgender (LGBT) Health. San Francisco (CA). 2001. Available at: http://www.glma.org/_data/n_0001/resources/live/HealthyCompanionDoc3.pdf. Accessed March 9, 2017.
13. Morrison MA, Morrison TG, Sager CL. Does body satisfaction differ between gay men and lesbian women and heterosexual men and women? A meta-analytic review. Body Image 2004;1(2):127–38.
14. Owens LK, Hughes TL, Owens-Nicholson D. The effects of sexual orientation on body image and attitudes about eating and weight. J Lesbian Stud 2003;7(1):15–33.
15. Alvy LM. Do lesbian women have a better body image? Comparisons with heterosexual women and model of lesbian-specific factors. Body Image 2013;10(4):524–34.
16. Koh AS, Ross LK. Mental health issues: a comparison of lesbian, bisexual and heterosexual women. J Homosex 2006;51(1):33–57.
17. Diemer EW, Grant JD, Munn-Chernoff MA, et al. Gender identity, sexual orientation, and eating-related pathology in a national sample of college students. J Adolesc Health 2014;57(2):144–9.
18. Vocks S, Stahn C, Loenser K, et al. Eating and body image disturbances in male-to-female and female-to-male transsexuals. Arch Sex Behav 2009;38(3):364–77.
19. Brown GR, Jones KT. Mental health and medical health disparities in 5135 transgender veterans receiving healthcare in the Veterans Health Administration: a case-control study. LGBT Heal 2016;3(2):122–31.
20. Bostwick WB, Boyd CJ, Hughes TL, et al. Dimensions of sexual orientation and the prevalence of mood and anxiety disorders in the United States. Am J Public Health 2010;100(3):468–75.
21. King M, Semlyen J, Tai SS, et al. A systematic review of mental disorder, suicide, and deliberate self harm in lesbian, gay and bisexual people. BMC Psychiatry 2008;8:70.
22. Cochran SD, Mays VM, Sullivan JG. Prevalence of mental disorders, psychological distress, and mental health services use among lesbian, gay, and bisexual adults in the United States. J Consult Clin Psychol 2003;71(1):53–61.
23. Gilman SE, Cochran SD, Mays VM, et al. Risk of psychiatric disorders among individuals reporting same-sex sexual partners in the national comorbidity survey. Am J Public Health 2001;91(6):933–9.
24. Gonzales G, Przedworski J, Henning-Smith C. Comparison of health and health risk factors between lesbian, gay, and bisexual adults and heterosexual adults in the United States. JAMA Intern Med 2016;176(9):1344–51.
25. Clements-Nolle K, Marx R, Mitchell Katz M, et al. Attempted suicide among transgender persons: the influence of gender-based discrimination and victimization. J Homosex 2006;51(3):53–69.
26. Hepp U, Kraemer B, Schnyder U, et al. Psychiatric comorbidity in gender identity disorder. J Psychosom Res 2005;58(3):259–61.
27. Nuttbrock L, Hwahng S, Bockting W, et al. Psychiatric impact of gender-related abuse across the life course of male-to-female transgender persons. J Sex Res 2010;47(1):12–23.

28. Khobzi Rotondi N, Bauer GR, Travers R, et al. Depression in male-to-female transgender Ontarians: results from the trans PULSE project. Can J Commun Ment Health 2011;30(2):113–33.
29. Budge SL, Adelson JL, Howard KAS. Anxiety and depression in transgender individuals: the roles of transition status, loss, social support, and coping. J Consult Clin Psychol 2013;81(3):545–57.
30. Hottes TS, Bogaert L, Rhodes AE, et al. Lifetime prevalence of suicide attempts among sexual minority adults by study sampling strategies: a systematic review and meta-analysis. Am J Public Health 2016;106(5):e1–12.
31. Blosnich JR, Nasuti LJ, Mays VM, et al. Suicidality and sexual orientation: characteristics of symptom severity, disclosure, and timing across the life course. Am J Orthopsychiatry 2016;86(1):69–78.
32. Cochran SD, Mays VM. Mortality risks among persons reporting same-sex sexual partners: evidence from the 2008 General Social Survey-National Death Index data set. Am J Public Health 2015;105(2):358–64.
33. Brown DC, Lariscy JT, Kalousová L. A comparison of mortality estimates from multiple nationally representative surveys and vital statistics data in the United States. In: Population Association of America Annual Meeting. Washington, DC, 2016. Available at: https://paa.confex.com/paa/2016/mediafile/ExtendedAbstract/Paper8033/Brown%20et%20al.%20(2016,%20Mortality%20Validation)%20PAA%20Final.pdf. Accessed March 9, 2017.
34. Carmel TC, Erickson-Schroth L. Mental health and the transgender population. Psychiatr Ann 2016;46(6):346–9.
35. Hoshiai M, Matsumoto Y, Sato T, et al. Psychiatric comorbidity among patients with gender identity disorder. Psychiatry Clin Neurosci 2010;64(5):514–9.
36. Liu RT, Mustanski B. Suicidal ideation and self-harm in lesbian, gay, bisexual, and transgender youth. Am J Prev Med 2012;42(3):221–8.
37. Case P, Austin B, Hunter DJ, et al. Sexual orientation, health risk factors, and physical functioning in the Nurses' Health Study II. J Womens Health 2004;13(9):1033–47.
38. Emory K, Kim Y, Buchting F, et al. Intragroup variance in lesbian, gay, and bisexual tobacco use behaviors: evidence that subgroups matter, notably bisexual women. Nicotine Tob Res 2016;18(6):1494–501.
39. Drabble L, Midanik LT, Trocki K. Reports of alcohol consumption and alcohol-related problems among homosexual, bisexual and heterosexual respondents: results from the 2000 National Alcohol Survey. J Stud Alcohol 2005;66(1):111–20.
40. McCabe SE, West BT, Hughes TL, et al. Sexual orientation and substance abuse treatment utilization in the United States: results from a national survey. J Subst Abuse Treat 2013;44(1):4–12.
41. McCabe SE, Hughes TL, Bostwick WB, et al. Sexual orientation, substance use behaviors and substance dependence in the United States. Addiction 2009;104(8):1333–45.
42. Cochran SD, Grella CE, Mays VM. Do substance use norms and perceived drug availability mediate sexual orientation differences in patterns of substance use? Results from the California Quality of Life Survey II. J Stud Alcohol Drugs 2012;73(4):675–85.
43. Benotsch EG, Zimmerman R, Cathers L, et al. Non-medical use of prescription drugs, polysubstance use, and mental health in transgender adults. Drug Alcohol Depend 2013;132(1–2):391–4.

44. Keuroghlian AS, Reisner SL, White JM, et al. Substance use and treatment of substance use disorders in a community sample of transgender adults. Drug Alcohol Depend 2015;152:139–46.
45. Risser JMH, Shelton A, McCurdy S, et al. Sex, drugs, violence, and HIV status among male-to-female transgender persons in Houston, Texas. Int J Transgenderism 2005;8(2–3):67–74.
46. Zimmerman RS, Benotsch EG, Shoemaker S, et al. Mediational models linking psychosocial context, mental health problems, substance use, and HIV risk behaviors in transgender women. Heal Psychol Behav Med 2015;3(1):379–90.
47. Lambda Legal. When health care isn't caring: Lamda Legal's survey on discrimination against LGBT people and people living with HIV. New York. 2010. Available at: http://www.lambdalegal.org/health-care-report. Accessed March 9, 2017.
48. Obedin-Maliver J, Goldsmith ES, Stewart L, et al. Lesbian, gay, bisexual, and transgender–related content in undergraduate medical education. JAMA 2011;306(9):971–7.
49. Drescher J. Gender diagnoses in the DSM and ICD. Psychiatr Ann 2016;46(6):350–4.
50. Substance Abuse and Mental Health Administration. Ending conversion therapy: supporting and affirming LGBTQ youth. Rockville (MD). 2015. Available at: http://store.samhsa.gov/product/Ending-Conversion-Therapy-Supporting-and-Affirming-LGBTQ-Youth/All-New-Products/SMA15-4928. Accessed March 9, 2017.

Update on Mental Health Aspects of Intimate Partner Violence

Donna Eileen Stewart, CM, MD, FRCPC[a,b,c,*],
Simone Natalie Vigod, MD, MSc, FRCPC[a,d]

KEYWORDS

- Intimate partner violence (IPV) • IPV prevalence • Risk factors • Adverse effects
- IPV identification and disclosure • IPV mental Health clinical management

KEY POINTS

- Intimate partner violence (IPV) occurs in more than one-third of American women and may cause serious physical and mental health sequelae.
- Physicians need to know the risk factors, how to assist disclosure of IPV, and how to safely respond to it.
- Psychiatrists must know the best short-term and long-term management and treatment of IPV mental health sequelae.

BACKGROUND

IPV is a serious global human rights and public health problem affecting individuals of all ages and walks of life. It can be perpetrated by a current or past partner in a heterosexual or same-sex relationship and at its core it is a means to control and dominate an abused partner. IPV may include acts of physical, sexual, or psychological

---

This is an update of an article that first appeared in the *Psychiatric Clinics of North America*, Volume 40, Issue 2, June 2017.
D.E. Stewart and S.N. Vigod both receive royalties from UpToDate Inc for authorship of materials related to depression and pregnancy. D.E. Stewart serves on the Duloxetine Pregnancy Registry (Eli Lilly) Medical Advisory Committee mandated by the FDA.
Funding Sources: None.
Conflict of Interest: Dr D.E. Stewart holds grants on this subject from Canadian Institutes of Health Research (PreVAiL Project, RDG99326) and the Public Health Agency of Canada (VEGA Project). Dr S.N. Vigod: None.
[a] University of Toronto, 200 Elizabeth Street, EN-7-229, Toronto, Ontario M5G 2C4, Canada; [b] Toronto General Hospital Research Institute, 200 Elizabeth Street, 7EN-229, Toronto, Ontario M5G 2C4, Canada; [c] Centre for Mental Health, University Health Network, 200 Elizabeth Street, 7EN-229, Toronto, Ontario M5G 2C4, Canada; [d] Women's College Hospital and Research Institute, 76 Grenville Street, Room 7234, Toronto, Ontario M5S 1B2, Canada
* Corresponding author. Toronto General Hospital, University Health Network, 200 Elizabeth Street, 7EN-229, Toronto, Ontario M5G 2C4, Canada.
E-mail address: donna.stewart@uhn.ca

Med Clin N Am 103 (2019) 735–749
http://dx.doi.org/10.1016/j.mcna.2019.02.010 medical.theclinics.com

aggression; stalking; and controlling behaviors and may cause physical, psychological, or sexual harm. Although both men and women may be victims, it is more common for men to perpetrate violence against women and for women's injuries to be more severe (including death) than those of men.[1]

IPV is the most common form of violence against women, with global lifetime prevalence rates ranging from 15% to 71%.[2] A US survey in 2011 found 36% of women and 29% of men reported lifetime IPV, with more serious injuries reported among women.[3] IPV is the leading cause of nonfatal injury to American women.[4]

Despite its high prevalence and serious health consequences IPV remains largely neglected as a physical and mental health priority.[5] Physicians and mental health professionals need to be knowledgeable about IPV and its mental health sequelae.[5,6] This article includes IPV background, definitions, prevalence, risk factors, adverse effects, identification, documentation, management across time, and conclusions, focusing on mental health.

DEFINITIONS

Several definitions of IPV exist, including one by the World Health Organization (WHO) as "behavior by an intimate partner that causes physical, sexual or psychological harm, including acts of physical aggression, sexual coercion, psychological abuse or controlling behaviors."[7] This article uses the Centers for Disease Control and Prevention (CDC) uniform definitions and some examples.[8]

Intimate Partner

"An intimate partner is a person with whom one has a close personal relationship that may be characterized by the partners' emotional connectedness, regular contact, ongoing physical contact and sexual behavior, identity as a couple, and familiarity and knowledge about each other's lives. The relationship need not involve all of these dimensions. Intimate partners may or may not be cohabiting. Intimate partners can be opposite or same sex. If the victim and the perpetrator have a child in common and a previous relationship but no current relationship, then by definition they fit into the category of former intimate partner."[8]

Intimate Partner Violence—Overall Definition

"Intimate partner violence includes physical violence, sexual violence, stalking and psychological aggression (including coercive tactics) by a current or former intimate partner (ie, spouse, boyfriend/girlfriend, dating partner, or ongoing sexual partner)."[8]

Physical violence

"Physical violence is defined as the intentional use of physical force with the potential for causing death, disability, injury, or harm"[8] (**Box 1**).

Sexual violence

"Sexual violence is defined as a sexual act that is committed or attempted by another person without freely given consent of the victim or against someone who is unable to consent or refuse"[8] (**Boxes 2** and **3**).

Penetration "Penetration involves physical insertion, however slight, of the penis into the vulva; contact between the mouth and the penis, vulva, or anus; or physical insertion of a hand, finger, or other object into the anal or genital opening of another person."[8]

Stalking

"A pattern of repeated, unwanted, attention and contact that causes fear or concern for one's own safety or the safety of someone else (eg, family member, close friend)"[8] (**Box 4**).

Box 1
Some examples of physical violence

Scratching
Pushing
Shoving
Throwing
Grabbing
Biting
Choking
Shaking
Hair pulling
Slapping
Punching
Hitting
Burning
Use of weapon
Use of restraints or body size/strength
Coercing others to perpetrate violence

Data from Breiding MJ, Basile KC, Smith SG, et al. Intimate partner violence surveillance: uniform definitions and recommended data elements, version 2.0. Atlanta (GA): National Center for Injury Prevention and Control, Centers for Disease Control and Prevention; 2015. Available at: http://www.cdc.gov/violenceprevention/pdf/intimatepartnerviolence.pdf. Accessed January 16, 2019.

Box 2
Some examples of sexual violence

- Completed or attempted forced penetration of victim
- Alcohol/drug-facilitated sexual acts
- Victim made to engage in sexual acts with someone
- Victim pressured verbally or through intimidation or misuse of authority to consent/acquiesce
- Unwanted sexual contact (eg, intentional touching)
- Noncontact unwanted sexual experiences (eg, sending sexual photos and harassment)

Data from Breiding MJ, Basile KC, Smith SG, et al. Intimate partner violence surveillance: uniform definitions and recommended data elements, version 2.0. Atlanta (GA): National Center for Injury Prevention and Control, Centers for Disease Control and Prevention; 2015. Available at: http://www.cdc.gov/violenceprevention/pdf/intimatepartnerviolence.pdf. Accessed January 16, 2019.

Box 3
Some sexual violence tactics

- Use or threat of physical force toward victim
- Administering alcohol or drugs to victim
- Victim is unable to provide consent due to incapacitation
- Exploitation of vulnerability (eg, immigration status, disability, and sexual orientation)
- Intimidation
- Misuse of authority
- Economic coercion (eg, bartering of sex for basic goods)
- Degradation (eg, insulting or humiliating victim)
- Fraud (eg, lies or misrepresentation of perpetrator's identity)
- Continual verbal pressure
- False promises by perpetrator (eg, promising marriage or to stay in the relationship)
- Nonphysical threats (eg, threats to end a relationship or spread rumors)

Data from Breiding MJ, Basile KC, Smith SG, et al. Intimate partner violence surveillance: uniform definitions and recommended data elements, version 2.0. Atlanta (GA): National Center for Injury Prevention and Control, Centers for Disease Control and Prevention; 2015. Available at: http://www.cdc.gov/violenceprevention/pdf/intimatepartnerviolence.pdf. Accessed January 16, 2019.

Box 4
Some examples of stalking

- Repeated and unwanted phone calls, voice/threat messages, pages, hang-ups
- Repeated and unwanted emails, instant messages, or through Web sites (eg, Facebook)
- Leaving unwanted cards, letters, flowers, or presents
- Watching or following from a distance
- Spying with a listening device, camera, or global positioning system
- Showing up in places (eg, home, work, and school) against victim's wishes
- Leaving strange or potentially threatening items for victim to find
- Sneaking into victim's home or car and doing things to scare victim
- Damaging victim's personal property, pets, or belongings
- Harming or threatening to harm victim's pet
- Making threats to physically harm victim

Data from Breiding MJ, Basile KC, Smith SG, et al. Intimate partner violence surveillance: uniform definitions and recommended data elements, version 2.0. Atlanta (GA): National Center for Injury Prevention and Control, Centers for Disease Control and Prevention; 2015. Available at: http://www.cdc.gov/violenceprevention/pdf/intimatepartnerviolence.pdf. Accessed January 16, 2019.

Psychological aggression
"Use of verbal and non-verbal communication with the intent to: (a) harm another person mentally or emotionally, and/or (b) exert control over another person"[8] (**Box 5**).

PREVALENCE

There are many challenges to obtaining accurate IPV prevalence figures. These include social barriers due to guilt and shame of asking about or disclosing

Box 5
Some examples of psychological aggression

- Expressive aggression (eg, name calling, humiliation, and degradation)
- Coercive control (eg, limiting access to money, friends, and family; excessive monitoring of a person's whereabouts and communications; monitoring or interfering with electronic communication threats to harm self; and threats to harm a loved one or possession)
- Threat of physical or sexual violence (eg, use of words, gestures, or weapons when victim is either unwilling or unable to consent)
- Control of reproductive or sexual health (eg, refusal to use birth control; coerced abortion)
- Exploitation of victim's vulnerability (eg, immigration status, disability, and undisclosed sexual orientation)
- Exploitation of perpetrator's vulnerability (eg, perpetrator's use of real or perceived disability, immigration status to control victim's choices or limit victim's options)
- Gaslighting (ie, mind games) — presenting false information to victims to cause them doubt about their memory and perception.

Data from Breiding MJ, Basile KC, Smith SG, et al. Intimate partner violence surveillance: uniform definitions and recommended data elements, version 2.0. Atlanta (GA): National Center for Injury Prevention and Control, Centers for Disease Control and Prevention; 2015. Available at: http://www.cdc.gov/violenceprevention/pdf/intimatepartnerviolence.pdf. Accessed January 16, 2019.

information about this sensitive topic, fear of repercussions, and lack of training of staff about how to ask. Financial or emotional dependence on the abuser, or fears about child custody or immigration status, may also be deterrents.[5] Data sources, such as police or justice reports, hospital or health records, and survey information, all underestimate IPV prevalence because many victims do not disclose or report.[5]

The US National Intimate Partner and Sexual Violence Survey under the CDC initiated a process to promote consistency in terminology and data collection that has assisted in regular updates about IPV prevalence.[8,9]

Overall, approximately 1 in 2 women experience lifetime psychological aggression, 1 in 3 physical violence, and 1 in 10 sexual violence or stalking by an intimate partner (**Table 1**).[9]

The WHO Global Status Report on Violence Prevention across the world, reported 1 in 2 women having been a victim of physical or sexual violence by her intimate partner during her lifetime.[10] The WHO Demographic and Health Surveys of 15 countries reported physical abuse during pregnancy ranging from 2% to 13.5%.[11] IPV occurs in all countries but differences in definition and methodology have resulted in difficulties in comparison. WHO conducted a 10-country survey of 24,097 women using comparable methodology, however, and found a reported prevalence of physical or sexual partner violence (or both) varied from 15% to 71% (lifetime) and 4% to 54% (past 12 months). In all but 1 setting, women were at far greater risk of physical or sexual violence by a partner than by other person.[12]

RISK FACTORS: A PUBLIC HEALTH MODEL

Past work on the risk factors associated with IPV tended to focus on the perpetrator or victim, but this resulted in a restricted view. A public health approach espoused by the WHO resulted in an ecological framework that views IPV as the outcome of interaction among many factors at 4 levels—individual, relationship, community, and societal (**Fig. 1**). This framework treats the interaction between factors at the different levels with equal importance as those within a single level.[13]

Individual factors include, among others, a past history of child maltreatment; psychological or personality disorders; violent behavior; alcohol/substance abuse; physical, mental, or intellectual disability; youth and old age; limited education; low income; medical illness; recent migration; sexual or visible minority; and indigenous status.[13]

Relationship factors include marital discord, alcohol/drug abuse, violent parental conflict, poor parenting practices, low socioeconomic status, friends who engage in

Table 1
Intimate partner violence in women

	Lifetime (%)	Last 12 mo (%)
Sexual violence (rape)	8.8	0.8
Other forms of sexual violence	15.8	2.1
Physical violence	31.5	4.0
Serious physical violence	22.3	2.3
Stalking	9.2	2.4
Psychological aggression	47.1	14.2

Modified from Breiding MJ, Smith SG, Basile KC, et al. Prevalence and characteristics of sexual violence, stalking, and intimate partner violence victimization–national intimate partner and sexual violence survey, United States, 2011. MMWR Surveill Summ 2014;63(8):1–18. Available at: https://www.cdc.gov/mmwr/preview/mmwrhtml/ss6308a1.htm. Accessed January 16, 2019.

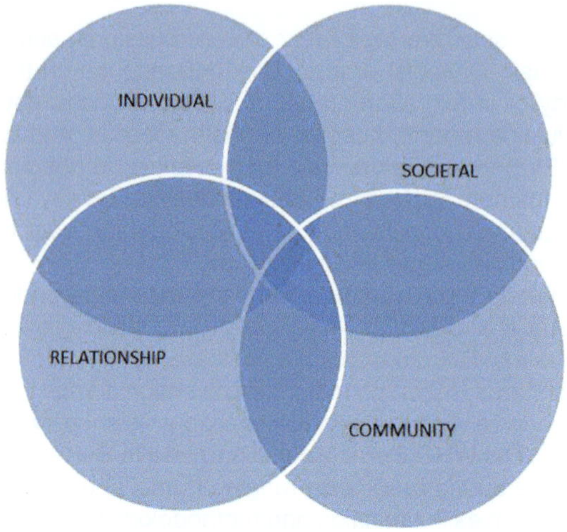

Fig. 1. The ecological framework. (*Adapted from* World Health Organization. World report on violence and health: summary. Geneva (Switzerland): WHO; 2002. p. 9. Available at: http://apps.who.int/iris/bitstream/10665/42512/1/9241545623_eng.pdf?ua=1.)

violence, poor or very different levels of education, need for overcontrol, negative attitudes toward women, history of child abuse or witnessing parental abuse, and having other sexual partners.[13]

Community factors include high crime levels, poverty, high unemployment, low social cohesion, high mobility, low opportunity, and lack of policies and services for women IPV victims (shelter, counseling, mental health, and social services).[13]

Social factors include gender inequality, cultural acceptance of IPV, restrictive laws on divorce, inheritance, and property rights, devaluation of women, normalizing or jokes about IPV, patriarchal laws, lack of legal and policy safeguards on IPV that are enforced, religious condoning of IPV, rapid social change, and many others.[13]

All these factors should be considered in discussing, preventing and treating IPV.

ADVERSE EFFECTS OF INTIMATE PARTNER VIOLENCE

IPV has widespread adverse effects on victims, perpetrators, families, social cohesion, and the economy. Its effects on a victim's physical and mental health can be profound.[14] A Kentucky study found 26% of all suicide cases between 2005–2015 were associated with intimate partner "problems", and 43% of these were also identified as IPV.[15]

In terms of physical health, the US Bureau of Justice in 2007 reported that 33% of female murder victims and 3% of male murder victims annually were killed by their partner or ex-partner.[16] A wide range of physical health sequelae may result in IPV victims, ranging from serious life-altering to temporary minor injuries (**Box 6**).[17] A narrative review of medical and social science literature found up to one-quarter of women attending sexual and reproductive health services reported reproductive control by others, mostly intimate partners.[18] Perinatal IPV may result in adverse health sequelae for both mother and developing fetus and infant.[19] A Japanese study found that IPV during pregnancy was significantly associated with later infant abuse and neglect.[20]

A multicountry WHO study of more than 24,000 women found an association between IPV and poor health, difficulty walking, difficulty with daily activities, memory loss, dizziness, and reproductive problems.[21] Apart from direct physical injuries, other chronic conditions may be associated with IPV through chronic stress or other mechanisms (**Box 7**).[17]

Box 6
Some physical health sequelae of intimate partner violence

Death

Brain injury

Fractures

Internal organ injuries

Burn disfigurements

Blindness/deafness

Contusions

Lacerations

Dental injuries

Functional gastrointestinal or musculoskeletal disorders

Chronic pain

HIV

Sexually transmitted diseases

Infertility

Miscarriage/fetal death

Unintended pregnancy

Sexual disorders

Pregnancy/fetal complications

Data from Centers for Disease Control and Prevention (CDC). Injury prevention & control: Division of violence prevention. Intimate partner violence: consequences. 2015. Available at: http://www.cdc.gov/violenceprevention/intimatepartnerviolence/consequences.html. Accessed January 16, 2019.

Box 7
Some examples of health conditions associated with intimate partner violence

- Asthma
- Bladder and kidney infections
- Circulatory conditions
- Cardiovascular disease
- Fibromyalgia
- Chronic fatigue
- Irritable bowel syndrome
- Chronic pain syndromes
- Central nervous system disorders
- Gastrointestinal disorders
- Joint disease
- Migraines and headaches

From Centers for Disease Control and Prevention (CDC). Injury prevention & control: Division of Violence Prevention. Intimate partner violence: consequences. 2015. Available at: http://www.cdc.gov/violenceprevention/intimatepartnerviolence/consequences.html. Accessed January 16, 2019.

Box 8
Some psychological consequences of intimate partner violence for victims

IPV (sexual, physical, or psychological) can lead to various psychological consequences

- Anxiety
- Depression
- PTSD
- Psychosis
- Antisocial behavior
- Suicidal behavior/self-harm
- Low self-esteem
- Inability to trust others
- Sexual dysfunction
- Emotional detachment
- Sleep disturbances
- Flashbacks
- Replaying the assault in the mind
- Appetite disturbances

From Centers for Disease Control and Prevention (CDC). Injury prevention & control: Division of Violence Prevention. Intimate partner violence: consequences. 2015. Available at: http://www.cdc.gov/violenceprevention/intimatepartnerviolence/consequences.html. Accessed January 16, 2019.

Physicians and mental health professionals, may see a wide range of psychological adverse sequelae.

There is also an increase in risky health behaviors, such as unsafe sex, unsafe diets, smoking, and alcohol and drug abuse (**Box 8**).

Although it is often not discussed (or inquired about), the prevalence of IPV in both ambulatory and hospitalized psychiatric patients is more than 30%.[22] A systematic review and meta-analysis (41 studies) found higher risks of adult IPV in women with

Box 9
Some social/economic costs of intimate partner violence

- Societal isolation
- Loss of usual activities
- School nonattendance
- Homelessness
- Work nonattendance/unemployment
- Poor role modeling for children
- Difficulty caring for children
- Worse quality of life

From Centers for Disease Control and Prevention (CDC). Injury prevention & control: Division of Violence Prevention. Intimate partner violence: consequences. 2015. Available at: http://www.cdc.gov/violenceprevention/intimatepartnerviolence/consequences.html. Accessed January 16, 2019.

depressive disorders (odds ratio [OR] 2.77), anxiety disorders (OR 4.08), and posttraumatic stress disorder (PTSD) (OR 7.34) compared with women without mental disorders.[23]

There may also be social and economic costs to IPV. On average, IPV victims make twice as many medical visits and 8 times as many mental health visits as other women. It has been estimated that IPV is as serious a cause of death and disability as cancer.[13] The CDC estimated a total cumulative cost of IPV to be more than $8 billion annually in the United States (**Box 9**).[17]

IDENTIFICATION AND DISCLOSURES

Controversy exists about the effectiveness of routine IPV screening in health care. Although the US Preventive Services Task Force, American Congress of Obstetricians and Gynecologists, US Department of Health and Human Services, and Affordable Care Act all recommend that IPV screening and counseling should be a core part of women's preventive health visits and at periodic intervals,[24] a Cochrane review of 8 studies involving more than 10,000 women concluded that there is insufficient evidence to justify universal IPV screening in a health care setting.[25] Due to the high prevalence of mental health sequelae associated with IPV, however, the US Substance Abuse and Mental Health Services Administration (SAMHSA) recommends physicians and mental health professionals practice a "trauma-informed" model of care for all patients (**Box 10**).[26]

Box 10
Trauma-informed model of care

- Program realizes widespread impact of IPV
- Recognizes stages and symptoms of trauma in clients and staff
- Integrates trauma knowledge in policies, procedures, and practices
- Actively seeks to avoid retraumatization
- Enforces principles of safety, trustworthiness, and transparency
- Models peer support, collaboration, mutuality, and empowerment
- Incorporates voice and choice, cultural, historical, and gender issues

Data from Substance Abuse and Mental Health Services Administration (SAMHSA). Trauma-informed approach and trauma-specific interventions. Available at: http://www.samhsa.gov/nctic/trauma-interventions. Accessed January 16, 2019.

Victims may not disclose out of embarrassment, fear, shame, or censure. It is often takes time for victims to decide to leave their partner, and they often go through several abusive episodes before leaving. Accordingly, questions about why victims do not leave their partners may be seen as unsupportive and judgmental. IPV victims want their health care providers to listen, express concern, and be empathic, nonjudgmental, and supportive.[27]

Case finding for IPV includes appropriately tailored questions about how disputes with a partner are resolved and feeling of safety at home (**Box 11**). These discussions must occur in a safe, private, confidential setting without the partner. Local laws often require reporting of IPV to child welfare authorities if children are victims or witnesses and, if this is the case, women should be told this before disclosure.[5] Although IPV is a crime in most jurisdictions, reporting (without child exposure) is usually not required

Box 11
Some possible intimate partner violence disclosure questions

- I'd like to ask about a sensitive personal issue.
- How are disputes with your partner resolved?
- It's important for me to understand my patient's safety in close relationships.
- Do you feel safe in your current or previous relationships?
- Have you ever been physically threatened or harmed by your partner or ex-partner?
- Sometimes partners or ex-partners use physical force—Is this happening to you?
- Have you felt humiliated or emotionally harmed by your partner or ex-partner?
- Have you ever been forced to have any kind of sexual activity by your partner or ex-partner?
- Do you feel your partner overcontrols you in your relationships with family or friends or in financial matters?

Adapted from Stewart DE, Vigod S, Riazantseva E. New developments in intimate partner violence and management of its mental health sequelae. Curr Psychiatry Rep 2016;18:4; with permission.

and should be a women's choice if not mandated because it may increase the victim's danger. It is important, however, to make inquiries about whether it is safe to return home and to help arrange practical supports and services, including a safety plan in the setting of acute risk. Regardless of the management plan, timely follow-up for ongoing monitoring and care should be arranged.

DOCUMENTATION

Because a medical record may be used in subsequent legal proceedings, it is vital that it be accurate and complete. It is useful to use a victim's own words in quotation marks. Details of the history, circumstances, chronology, signs, symptoms, evidence, and names of witnesses (if any) should be recorded. Measurement and full description of injuries are required. A dated body diagram or photograph (with the victim's permission) of any visible injuries can assist in documentation. Mental health signs and symptoms should be noted.[5] Separation of facts and opinions should be clear. If the abuse is reported, details of the report and receiving authority should be recorded.

PREVENTION OF MENTAL HEALTH SEQUELAE

Factors that increase risk for the development of mental health sequelae of trauma include biological predisposition to mental illness, prior history of psychosocial adversity, intensity and chronicity of the trauma, and posttrauma adversities, which in cases of IPV may include life stress, such as financial problems or loss of social support systems related to the ongoing IPV, disclosure about the IPV, or action to remove oneself from an abusive relationship.[28] Yet, it remains difficult to know how these factors will interact to predict the nature and intensity of mental health symptoms for any given individual experiencing IPV, creating challenges for efforts to prevent the mental health sequelae of IPV. In terms of prevention, however, social support has been identified as a key protective factor against the development of mental health sequelae of IPV. Therefore, in the acute phase after identification of IPV, clinicians should engage in efforts to mobilize social supports and facilitate referrals to legal, medical, and psychosocial services as appropriate. These involve not only obtaining appropriate referrals but also educating victims about the mental health symptoms that may emerge with trauma and that it is normal to need support.[29] Individuals experiencing high levels of distressing symptoms, such as anxiety, hyperarousal, irritability, sleep disturbance, and re-experiencing phenomenon, may benefit acutely from learning grounding strategies designed to help calm some of the physiologic arousal symptoms and focus on the present (not past or future). When symptoms are not manageable with nonpharmacological strategies, a short-term prescription for an antianxiety medication, such as a benzodiazepine, may be appropriate to allow for sleep and periods of temporary symptom relief.[29] A Cochrane review evaluated 9 randomized controlled trials of pharmacologic interventions designed to prevent the onset of PTSD after acute trauma, such as accidents, work trauma, and assault, finding some evidence for efficacy of hydrocortisone (3 of 4 trials) but not for escitalopram, temazepam, or gabapentin.[30] This finding requires replication before it becomes standard clinical practice. Whether hydrocortisone could prevent PTSD onset in an individual exposed to chronic trauma, as is often the case in IPV, is unknown.

TREATMENT

Over the past several years, there has been an increasing focus on having a trauma-informed model of mental health treatment, regardless of whether the mental health presentation is an anxiety, depressive, or stressor-related disorder and/or whether it includes other comorbidities, such as substance abuse and eating disorder. According to SAMHSA, trauma-specific interventions also recognize a survivor's need to be respected, informed, and empowered.[26] This helps ensure that interventions are not experienced as a form of revictimization and that the survivor is engaged in long-term treatment planning.[26] Several psychological interventions have been specifically evaluated in individuals with chronic symptoms of PTSD, one of the most common sequelae of IPV. These include trauma-focused (TF)–cognitive behavior therapy (CBT) and eye-movement desensitization and reprocessing (EMDR),[31] In TF-CBT, treatment is focused specifically on exposure to the traumatic event, either imagined or in vivo exposure to the traumatic situation, and on challenging maladaptive thoughts and behaviors related to the event and its consequences. EMDR involves desensitization to the traumatic experience through standardized procedures, where spontaneous associations of traumatic images, cognitions, feelings, and body sensations are paired with repetitive eye movements or other bilateral stimulation procedures. A Cochrane review found both TF-CBT and EMDR seem more effective than usual care in reducing symptoms of PTSD and that they may be superior to non–TF-CBT and other nonspecific therapies over the longer term.[31] Among individuals with comorbid substance use disorders, TF psychological treatment may be more effective at reducing both PTSD and substance use disorder symptoms[32] than non-TF therapy and usual care. A systematic review by the US Agency for Healthcare Research and Quality found psychotherapies with high strength of evidence for PTSD included cognitive behavioral therapy-exposure (CBT-E) and CBT—mixed treatments. Moderate strength of evidence was found for cognitive processing therapy (CPT), cognitive therapy (CT), eye movement desensitization and reprocessing (EMDR) and narrative exposure therapy (NET).[33]

According to a systematic review by the US Agency for Healthcare Research and Quality, pharmacotherapies with at least a moderate strength of evidence to support their efficacy in the relief of PTSD symptoms are fluoxetine, paroxetine, and venlafaxine.[33,34] One randomized controlled trial found EMDR and fluoxetine treatment comparable with respect to short-term outcomes, but its results

Box 12
Psychological and pharmacologic interventions with most evidence for posttraumatic stress disorder treatment

Psychological treatments

- High strength of evidence: CBT-E, CBT-mixed treatments
- Moderate strength of evidence: CPT, CT, EMDR, NET

Medication treatments

- Moderate strength of evidence: Antidepressants (fluoxetine, paroxetine and venlafaxine)
- Lower strength of evidence: Prazosin, sertraline, topiramate, antipsychotics (olanzapine, risperidone)

Data from Hoffman V, Middleton JC, Feltner C, et al. Psychological and Pharmacological Treatments for Adults With Posttraumatic Stress Disorder: A Systematic Review Update. Comparative Effectiveness Review No. 207. (Prepared by the RTI International–University of North Carolina at Chapel Hill Evidence-based Practice Center under Contract No. 290-2015-00011-I for AHRQ and PCORI.) AHRQ Publication No. 18-EHC011-EF. PCORI Publication No. 2018-SR-01. Rockville (MD): Agency for Healthcare Research and Quality; May 2018.

suggested that response to EMDR may be more sustained at 6-month follow-up.[35] Physicians who are not trained in the use of psychotherapies or pharmacotherapies should refer to appropriate mental health professionals, usually psychiatrists (**Box 12**).[33]

The treatment of perpetrators of IPV is a vital issue. If there is an underlying diagnosis such as depression, anxiety, psychoses, substance abuse or brain disease, this should be addressed, however, such conditions are relatively rare in IPV perpetrators. Personality disorders, anger and control issues, childhood exposure to abuse, hypermasculinity, denial, and dysfunctional social attitudes are more common.[36] Several batterer intervention programs exist with low to modest results.[37,38] Dysfunctional thinking in IPV perpetrators has led to the development of cognitive behavioral therapy programs. A 2011 Cochrane review of the effectiveness of cognitive behavioral group therapy on men's behaviour toward their female partner who they had abused was updated to 2018, and found insufficient evidence to confirm a positive effect, as had been shown in 2011.[39] Clearly more work is required to develop effective treatment for IPV perpetrators.

SUMMARY

IPV is a common occurrence and is particularly prevalent among women presenting with mental health concerns, including depression, anxiety, PTSD, substance use, eating disorders, and a host of psychosomatic conditions that may be seen by physicians and mental health professionals. We can improve patient outcomes by knowing the risk factors for IPV, how to assist in disclosure, and how to safely respond with practical, psychoeducational, and therapeutic interventions within a trauma-informed framework. For psychiatrists and other appropriately trained physicians and mental health professionals both psychological and pharmacologic therapies may be effective at minimizing mental health aspects of IPV, with emerging evidence that psychotherapies, such as CBT-enhanced therapies and EMDR, may be more effective than usual care or other therapies in the treatment of chronic PTSD symptoms and may produce a more sustained response to treatment compared with pharmacotherapeutic strategies alone.

REFERENCES

1. Stewart DE, Vigod S, Riazantseva E. New developments in intimate partner violence and management of its mental health sequelae. Curr Psychiatry Rep 2016;18:4.
2. World Health Organization. Responding to intimate partner violence and sexual violence against women: WHO clinical and policy guidelines. Geneva (Switzerland): WHO; 2013. Available at: http://apps.who.int/iris/bitstream/10665/85240/1/9789241548595_eng.pdf?ua=1. Accessed January 16, 2019.
3. Black M, Basile K, Breiding M, et al. The National Intimate Partner and Sexual Violence Survey (NISVS): 2010 Summary Report. Atlanta (GA); 2011. Available at: https://www.cdc.gov/violenceprevention/pdf/nisvs_report2010-a.pdf. Accessed January 16, 2019.
4. Tjaden P, Thoennes N. Extent, nature, and consequences of intimate partner violence. Washington, DC; 2002. Available at: https://www.ncjrs.gov/pdffiles1/nij/181867.pdf. Accessed January 16, 2019.
5. Stewart DE, MacMillan H, Wathen N. Intimate partner violence. Can J Psychiatry 2013;58:1–15.
6. World Health Organization, Pan American Health Organization. Strengthening the Capacity of Health-Care Providers to Address Violence against Women. WHO and PAHO Expert Meeting on Curricula Development. Washington, DC, September 30, 2015.
7. World Health Organization. Health care for women subjected to intimate partner violence or sexual violence: a clinical handbook. 2014. Available at: http://apps.who.int/iris/bitstream/10665/136101/1/WHO_RHR_14.26_eng.pdf?ua=1. Accessed January 16, 2019.
8. Breiding M, Basile K, Smith S, et al. Intimate partner violence surveillance: uniform definitions and recommended data elements version 2.0. National Center for Injury Prevention and Control, Centers for Disease Control and Prevention. Atlanta (GA); 2015. Available at: http://www.cdc.gov/violenceprevention/pdf/intimatepartnerviolence.pdf. Accessed January 16, 2019.
9. Breiding M, Smith S, Basile K, et al. Prevalence and characteristics of sexual violence, stalking, and intimate partner violence victimization–national intimate partner and sexual violence survey, United States, 2011. MMWR Surveill Summ 2014;63(8):1–18. Available at: http://www.ncbi.nlm.nih.gov/pubmed/25188037. Accessed January 16, 2019..
10. World Health Organization, United Nations Development Programme, United Nations Office on Drugs and Crime. The Global Status Report on Violence Prevention 2014. Available at: http://www.who.int/violence_injury_prevention/violence/status_report/2014/en/. Accessed January 16, 2019.
11. Devries KM, Kishor S, Johnson H, et al. Intimate partner violence during pregnancy: analysis of prevalence data from 19 countries. Reprod Health Matters 2010;18:158–70.
12. Garcia-Moreno C, Jansen HAFM, Ellsberg M, et al. Prevalence of intimate partner violence: findings from the WHO multi-country study on women's health and domestic violence. Lancet 2006;368:1260–9.
13. World Health Organization. World report on violence and health: summary. Geneva (Switzerland): WHO; 2002. Available at: http://apps.who.int/iris/bitstream/10665/42512/1/9241545623_eng.pdf?ua=1. Accessed July 5, 2016.
14. Campbell JC. Health consequences of intimate partner violence. Lancet 2002;359:1331–6.

15. Brown S, Seals J. Intimate partner problems and suicide: are we missing the violence? J Inj Violence Res 2019;11(1).
16. Fox J, Zawitz M. Homicide trends in the United States: intimate homicide. Washington, DC; 2007. Available at: http://www.bjs.gov/index.cfm?ty=pbdetail&iid=966. Accessed July 5, 2016.
17. Centers for Disease Control and Prevention. Injury prevention & control: division of violence prevention. Intimate partner violence: consequences. 2015. Available at: http://www.cdc.gov/violenceprevention/intimatepartnerviolence/consequences.html. Accessed July 5, 2016.
18. Rowlands S, Walker S. Reproductive control by others: means, perpetrators and effects. BMJ Sex Reprod Health 2019;45(1):61–7.
19. Han A, Stewart DE. Maternal and fetal outcomes of intimate partner violence associated with pregnancy in the Latin American and Caribbean region. Int J Gynaecol Obstet 2014;124:6–11.
20. Kita S, Chan KL, Tobe H, et al. A follow-up study on the continuity and spillover effects of intimate partner violence during pregnancy on postnatal child abuse. J Interpers Violence 2019 Jan 10:886260518821460.
21. Ellsberg M, Jansen HAFM, Heise L, et al. Intimate partner violence and women's physical and mental health in the WHO multi-country study on women's health and domestic violence: an observational study. Lancet 2008;371:1165–72.
22. Oram S, Trevillion K, Feder G, et al. Prevalence of experiences of domestic violence among psychiatric patients: systematic review. Br J Psychiatry 2013;202:94–9.
23. Trevillion K, Oram S, Feder G, et al. Experiences of domestic violence and mental disorders: a systematic review and meta-analysis. PLoS One 2012;7:e51740.
24. Agency for Healthcare Research and Quality, Rockville M. Intimate partner violence screening. 2015. Available at: http://www.ahrq.gov/professionals/prevention-chronic-care/healthier-pregnancy/preventive/partnerviolence.html. Accessed January 16, 2019.
25. O'Doherty L, Hegarty K, Ramsay J, et al. Screening women for intimate partner violence in healthcare settings. Cochrane Database Syst Rev 2015;(7). CD007007. Available at: http://www.cochrane.org/CD007007/BEHAV_screening-women-intimate-partner-violence-healthcare-settings. Accessed January 16, 2019.
26. Substance Abuse and Mental Health Services Administration. Trauma-informed approach and trauma-specific interventions | SAMHSA. Available at: http://www.samhsa.gov/nctic/trauma-interventions. Accessed January 16, 2019.
27. Feder GS, Hutson M, Ramsay J, et al. Women exposed to intimate partner violence: expectations and experiences when they encounter health care professionals: a meta-analysis of qualitative studies. Arch Intern Med 2006;166:22–37.
28. Brewin C, Andrews B, Valentine J. Meta-analysis of risk factors for posttraumatic stress disorder in trauma-exposed adults. J Consult Clin Psychol 2000;68(5): 748–66.
29. Vigod S, Stewart DE. Psychiatric management of victims of intimate partner and sexual violence. In: Tasman A, Kay J, Lieberman JA, et al, editors. Psychiatry. 4th edition. Chichester (UK): John Wiley & Sons, Ltd; 2015. p. 2533–48.
30. Amos T, Stein DJ, Ipser JC. Pharmacological interventions for preventing post-traumatic stress disorder (PTSD). Cochrane Database Syst Rev 2014;(7):CD006239.
31. Bisson JI, Roberts NP, Andrew M, et al. Psychological therapies for chronic post-traumatic stress disorder (PTSD) in adults. Cochrane Database Syst Rev 2013;(12):CD003388.

32. Roberts NP, Roberts PA, Jones N, et al. Psychological therapies for post-traumatic stress disorder and comorbid substance use disorder. Cochrane Database Syst Rev 2016;(4):CD010204.
33. Hoffman V, Middleton JC, Feltner C, et al. Psychological and Pharmacological Treatments for Adults With Posttraumatic Stress Disorder: A Systematic Review Update. Comparative Effectiveness Review No. 207. (Prepared by the RTI International–University of North Carolina at Chapel Hill Evidence-based Practice Center under Contract No. 290-2015-00011-I for AHRQ and PCORI.) AHRQ Publication No. 18-EHC011-EF. PCORI Publication No. 2018-SR-01. Rockville (MD): Agency for Healthcare Research and Quality; 2018.
34. Jonas D, Cusack K, Forneris C, et al. Psychological and pharmacological treatments for adults with posttraumatic stress disorder (PTSD). Comp Eff Rev 2013;92.
35. van der Kolk BA, Spinazzola J, Blaustein ME, et al. A randomized clinical trial of eye movement desensitization and reprocessing (EMDR), fluoxetine, and pill placebo in the treatment of posttraumatic stress disorder: treatment effects and long-term maintenance. J Clin Psychiatry 2007;68:37–46.
36. Elklit A, Murphy S, Jacobsen C, et al. Clinical and personality disorders in a danish treatment-seeking sample of intimate partner violence perpetrators. Int J Offender Ther Comp Criminol 2018;62(11):3322–36.
37. Morrison PK, Hawker L, Cluss PA, et al. The challenges of working with men who perpetrate partner violence: perspectives and observations of experts who work with batterer intervention programs. J Interpers Violence 2018 Jun 1:886260518778258.
38. Voith LA, Logan-Greene P, Strodthoff T, et al. A paradigm shift in batterer intervention programming: a need to address unresolved trauma. Trauma Violence Abuse 2018 Jul 30:1524838018791268.
39. Nesset MB, Lara-Cabrera ML, Dalsbø TK, et al. Cognitive behavioural group therapy for male perpetrators of intimate partner violence: a systematic review. BMC Psychiatry 2019;19(1):11.

Update on Reproductive Rights and Women's Mental Health

Nada Logan Stotland, MD, MPH

KEYWORDS

• Reproductive rights • Women • Mental health • Barriers

KEY POINTS

- This article explores the origins of barriers to reproductive rights, the nature of these barriers, and their impact on women's mental health.
- Reproductive rights are essential to the recognition and treatment of women as human beings and citizens. Barriers to reproductive rights thus pose a grave danger to women's overall well-being.
- The most controversial relationship is between induced abortion and women's mental health. There is a solid body of evidence demonstrating the absence of negative effect.
- Barriers, misinformation, and coercion affecting contraceptive, abortion, and pregnancy care are an ongoing danger to women's mental health and to the well-being of their families.
- Mental health professionals are obligated to know the facts, apply them, and provide accurate information to protect women's health.

INTRODUCTION

The World Health Organization declares reproductive rights to be essential human rights and has issued many statements, manuals, and guidelines for the implementation of those rights.[1–4] The American Psychiatric Association has adopted a series of

---

This is an update of an article that first appeared in the *Psychiatric Clinics of North America*, Volume 40, Issue 2, June 2017.

Since this article was written, the New York Times, on Sunday, January 20th, 2019, published a 12-page Special Opinion Report covering the dangers to women's fundamental rights, both threatened and accomplished, of designating the fetus as a person. The report is titled "A Woman's Right;" authorship is credited to the Times' Editorial Board.

No commercial or financial conflicts of interest.

Disclosure: Neither the author nor any member of her immediate family has any financial or administrative interest in the topics discussed in this article. She has served on the Board of Physicians for Reproductive Choice and Health. She has testified in opposition to restrictive abortion laws in the United States Congress and in several states. She accepted no remuneration for this testimony.

Department of Psychiatry, Rush University, 5511 South Kenwood Avenue, Chicago, Illinois 60637-1713, USA

E-mail address: nada.stotland@gmail.com

Med Clin N Am 103 (2019) 751–766
http://dx.doi.org/10.1016/j.mcna.2019.02.006 **medical.theclinics.com**

policies recognizing reproductive rights and advocating against laws and other barriers to their realization.[5–9]

Women's reproductive rights are not limited to access to contraception and abortion. Reproductive rights compass the status of women as citizens. The many laws and court decisions restricting contraception and abortion, and forcing interventions on pregnant women, in the United States and elsewhere, deny women rights as do no other health-related laws and decisions.

In the United States, no person can be legally forced to contribute 1 drop of blood, even to save the life of a scientific genius, virtuoso musician, or world leader. Nevertheless, pregnant women may be forced to undergo surgical procedures deemed to be necessary for the well-being of fetuses: potential persons.[10] Laws limiting access to contraception and abortion, permitting forced interventions during pregnancy, and criminalizing personal behaviors of pregnant women are demeaning to women. They are based on the premise that women do not understand their condition when pregnant, are unable to make considered decisions about their pregnancies, and that their lives are less important than those of embryos. Laws that mandate specific procedures or force physicians to provide specific misinformation to pregnant patients contravene medical ethics, interfere with the patient–physician relationship, and thus deprive pregnant women of their right to ethical, science-based medical care.[11]

This article does not use the term 'prolife,' coined by antiabortion groups and, unfortunately, adopted almost universally in public discourse. Words are powerful.[12] Of course, life is precious. But the term 'prolife' limits the desired protection of 'life' to the fertilized egg, embryo, and fetus. It does not compass, for example, the abolition of the death penalty in the criminal justice system. It does not include responsibility for a child born to an unwilling or unprepared mother, or for any human being once it is born. It makes the pregnant woman's life of no consequence. This article is based on reviews of the scientific literature, and information about laws, legal cases, and other events. Nevertheless, it must reflect the author's deep concern about the disregard for and hostility toward women reflected in the attacks on women's reproductive rights. Following are introductory examples. As this article is being written, Roman Catholic hospitals are not permitted to perform abortions even when there is no hope of extrauterine life for the fetus and the pregnant woman's life is acutely threatened by the pregnancy.[13,14] Currently, a woman is in prison for attempting suicide while pregnant.[10] Michael Pence is vice president of the United States. As Governor of the State of Indiana, Mr. Pence signed into law, in 2016, an act forbidding abortion for genetic defects, making the voluntary donation of fetal tissue a felony, and requiring that all "fetal remains," regardless of their origin or stage of gestation, be buried or cremated.[15]

This article addresses the history of reproductive rights, the current status of reproductive rights; the assumptions about and attitudes toward women reflected in those rights, or the absence of them; the impact of rights denied versus fulfilled on women's mental health; and both the scientific facts and the rampant misinformation about the impact of induced abortion on women's mental health. The article focuses on these issues in the United States, where they are problematic, public, and hotly contested. Although there is some controversy over women's right to contraceptives, the denial of rights mostly concerns emergency contraception (eg, levonorgestrel [Plan B]) and the rights of women during pregnancy.

In addition to the damages caused by the denial of reproductive rights to women in general, restrictions and requirements exacerbate the negative mental health concomitants of poverty, domestic violence, poor education, and racial discrimination.[1] The limitations differentially affect women in inverse relation to their socioeconomic status; it is poor women who are most vulnerable to unplanned and untenable pregnancies, and poor women who face the most barriers to ending those pregnancies.[16] With regard to abortion, there is considerable scientific evidence about its relationship to mental health. With regard to forced bodily intrusions and differential access, we must rely on our knowledge of the impact of injustice and abuse on mental well-being.[17–21]

HISTORY

The concept of reproductive rights is relatively new. Throughout history, women have been expected to marry. Within marriage, women were bound to submit to sexual intercourse and, thus, pregnancy. There were penalties for women who became pregnant outside of marriage.

Although effective contraception and safe abortion only became available in the mid-twentieth century, historical and anthropological studies reveal that contraception and abortion were attempted or practiced in a wide variety of times and places. Abortion techniques are described in Egyptian medical papyruses dating from 1700 BC. The Hippocratic Oath is often cited as evidence that abortion was forbidden in ancient Greece. In fact, the Hippocratic Oath is evidence that abortion was practiced in ancient Greece. Had it not been practiced, there would have been no need to mention it. A number of ancient medical or gynecologic texts describe abortifacient drugs, and ancient tools used for surgical abortions have been discovered.[22,23]

Women's magazines in the nineteenth century carried advertisements for purported abortifacients thinly disguised as menstrual or other remedies.[24] Historical texts seem to imply that herbal and other remedies were effective abortifacients, but no evidence was gathered, and no such effective method is now known. As far as we know, abortion was fraught with a high risk of physical pain, morbidity, and mortality until the advent of sterile technique, anesthesia, and access to both in fairly recent decades.

The popular BBC television series *Call the Midwife*, set in a low-income neighborhood in post World War II London, included an episode in which the impoverished, married, mother of several children desperately sought and underwent an abortion apparently induced by a local woman who administered some caustic substance. The woman's life was barely saved. Nevertheless, through her pain, the woman only cares about one thing: "Has it [the embryo] come away?" The fact is that neither civil laws, religious prohibitions, pain, and the very real fear of death prevent millions of women from attempting abortions. It is estimated that 56.3 million women worldwide per year have abortions and that well over 20,000 women per year who must resort to illegal, unsafe abortions die from them. The fact that abortion was practiced for millennia before it was safe, and that thousands of women worldwide die from unsafe abortions each year, in the twenty-first century, is testimony to the intensity, the desperation, with which women regard control of their procreative functions. Those who prohibit or limit abortion are therefore subjecting women, and the existing children and other dependents who need them, to mental and physical damage.

ABORTION METHODS AND SAFETY

Abortion can be accomplished medically, on an outpatient basis, using oral mifepristone to block the progesterone essential to the maintenance of the uterine lining, followed by misoprostol to induce contractions and empty the uterus. Years of experience with medical abortion have led experts to lessen the recommended dose, to widen the window of effectiveness, and to relax standards for observation. The process does not require anesthesia or the use of any medical facility. In an outpatient clinic, an early pregnancy can be terminated via suction or dilatation and evacuation (D and E), using local anesthesia. The advantage, as compared with medical abortion, is that the process is complete once the patient leaves the facility. Medical abortion causes some hours of cramping and bleeding, which are uncomfortable and inconvenient.

The data on the physical risks of abortion are clear. Abortion does not increase the risk of breast cancer or impair future fertility. Induced abortion is among the safest interventions in all of medicine. Abortion carries far less risk of physical and psychological morbidity and mortality than childbirth—the only alternative for the pregnant woman. Colonoscopy, a procedure strongly recommended for nearly universal application to adults, carries a 10 times greater risk of complications than abortion.[25]

RELIGION, HISTORY, AND ABORTION

Many Americans may mistakenly believe that abortion is forbidden by all religions. This is not true.[26] A blanket prohibition on abortion is not part of the ancient Judeo-Christian tradition. Traditional Judaism allowed for abortion at early stages of pregnancy, at least under some circumstances, including danger to the mother's health. Similar latitude exists in the Islamic tradition. The early Roman Catholic Church regarded abortion as acceptable until the fetus was considered to have a soul, as evidenced by its movements in utero as perceived by the mother: quickening. Current church doctrine, although forbidding abortion regardless of the circumstances, states that there is disagreement among theologians as to when the embryo becomes a person and is thus entitled to the protections due a person. Many non-Evangelical Protestant denominations, as well as non-Orthodox Jewish scholars, support latitude in abortion decisions. Although traditional Taoism, Buddhism, and Hinduism explicitly forbid abortion, abortion is widely practiced in India, China, and other countries espousing these faiths.[27]

ABORTION DEMOGRAPHICS

The Guttmacher Institute, New York City, gathers and makes available on its website (www.guttmacher.org) information relevant to contraception and abortion throughout the world. In the United States, 30% of women will have an abortion by age 45. Among women who have abortions:

- 75% are poor or have low income;
- 62% profess a religious affiliation;
- 59% already have a child;
- 60% are in their 20s;
- 12% are teens;
- 4% are minors;
- 39% are white;
- 28% black; and
- 25% Hispanic.

Women of various religions have abortions in percentages to their representation in society as a whole; that is, women who profess religions opposed to abortion have abortions just as often as those who do not profess such religions.[28,29]

BASIC REPRODUCTIVE KNOWLEDGE

The right to know is central to rights to reproductive health and health care. Many women cannot draw a substantially accurate representation of their reproductive systems. They do not know when, during their menstrual cycles, they are most fertile. Misinformation about conception and contraception is rife. Some adolescents believe that douching with a carbonated beverage can prevent pregnancy, that coitus interruptus prevents pregnancy, and/or that pregnancy cannot result from first intercourse.[30]

Unfortunately, much sex education—where there is sex education—in the United States is predicated on the misapprehension that the provision of information about sex encourages sexual activity. The United States government funds abstinence-only sex education, which has proved counterproductive. To encourage abstinence, the effectiveness of contraceptives is downplayed and the risks of contraceptives are exaggerated. The students are given no realistic approaches to their own sexuality, and those who do have intercourse are less likely to use contraception. Young women are not given information they need about their right to make their own decisions about sexual activity and assertiveness tools to enable them to effect that right.

REASONS FOR ABORTION

Women undergoing abortion report that they have chosen to terminate their pregnancies because of poverty, domestic violence, lack of other social supports, youth, and their need to complete their educations or establish their careers.[31] Lay people and professionals may assume that pregnancy would be a protection from interpersonal violence; in fact, pregnancy does not diminish, and may even increase, the incidence of violence against women. There are strong links between domestic violence and abortion; abusers may coerce women into intercourse, refuse or forbid the use of contraception, and inherently make the domestic situation dangerous for mother and child.[32–35]

MENTAL HEALTH OUTCOMES OF ABORTION

Mental health risks are the cited rationale for some restrictive laws regarding abortion. However, a review of the published evidence reveals several decades of consistently reassuring findings, including thorough literature reviews by the American Psychological Association and the Royal Colleges of Physicians, in contrast with a string of methodologically unacceptable papers claiming adverse psychiatric sequelae.[36–43] Poorly done studies compare the mental well-being of women who have abortions with that of women who go on to deliver or with the general population of women. They fail to recognize that the circumstances of individuals undergoing abortions are not comparable either with the general population or with women who opt to continue their pregnancies. They do not provide baseline data about the mental health of the woman before the abortion. They do not take the circumstances that occasioned the decision for abortion into account.[44,45] The reasons women decide to abort are all mental health risk factors—poverty, lack of social supports, domestic violence, rape, incest, heavy ongoing responsibilities, lack of education—and preexisting mental illness. The strongest predictor of a woman's mental health after an abortion is her mental health before an abortion.[46] Abortion may be associated with alcohol and substance abuse, suicidality, depression, and anxiety, but it does not cause them. Difficulty obtaining an abortion for whatever reason increases a woman's stress, as does exposure to clinic demonstrators, not to mention criminal attacks on abortion facilities and clinic staff.[47]

The publication of the studies claiming to have found negative mental health effects of abortion has led to consternation in the scientific community and the publication of reanalyses pointing out gross methodological errors, invalidating the conclusions, and ultimately resulting in disavowal of 1 paper by the editors of the journal that published it.[48,49] Nevertheless, misinformation and misdirection are rampant.[50,51] A Google search on abortion undertaken in June 2016 quickly led to a website called

TeenBreak, which informs the hapless pregnant teen, or her adult advisers, that abortion causes depression, suicidality, and other dire mental health outcomes. Many of the resources listed at the top of such searches are actually disguised antiabortion centers. The federal government, and some states, continue to fund so-called 'pregnancy crisis centers,' which advertise help and choice for pregnant women, but actually exist to deter women from having abortions. They provide misinformation and antiabortion persuasion. Some offer free ultrasound imaging and deliberately delay conveying the results to the pregnant woman so that it will be too late for her to go to an abortion facility.

The decision to terminate a pregnancy may be easy or difficult, depending on a woman's circumstances and beliefs. After abortion, women experience a wide variety of feelings: guilt, sadness, and, most prominently, relief. These feelings must not be confused with psychiatric disorders; they evolve over time and depend on ensuing circumstances.[52]

PSYCHOSOCIAL UNDERPINNINGS AND PUBLIC MANIFESTATIONS OF OPPOSITION TO ABORTION

Strong feelings about mothers in general, and one's own mother, are core elements of human psychology. For a young child, its mother is the most powerful person on earth. That power can be reassuring, but also terrifying. Anxiety about one's own wantedness may give rise to objections to abortion. Some groups representing people with disabilities oppose abortion because they believe that aborting fetuses with genetic or other defects is evidence that their own lives are not considered worthwhile. At worst, abortion is felt to be the manifestation of women's murderous wishes toward their children. Abortion represents, for some who oppose it, the rejection of women's submissive and maternal role, thus threatening both the males dominant in society and the women who feel valued only on the basis of motherhood and the fulfillment of religious requirements that women submit to their husbands.

Unplanned pregnancy in a sexual partner can arouse a wide variety of psychological reactions in a man. He may be proud of his virility. He may be pleased by the prospect of having a child, and with this partner. If his partner had led him to believe that a pregnancy was not possible, he may feel tricked and trapped. He may feel guilty for conceiving the pregnancy and forcing his partner either to undergo an abortion or give birth to a baby. If the pregnancy is unwelcome to him, but his partner opts to remain pregnant, he may feel obligated to a lifetime in the relationship and as a father. If his partner opts to terminate the pregnancy, where that is possible, he may feel helpless to protect, and deprived of, his potential child.

Attitudes toward women's sexuality color beliefs and attitudes toward contraception and abortion. Although women's ability to force men into sexual intercourse is limited by sexual anatomy and physiology, as well as the gender differential in physical strength, women have been, and continue to be, held accountable for male sexual aggression. It was Eve who ate the apple, sexually seduced Adam, and occasioned their ouster from the Garden of Eden. Orthodox Judaism, Hinduism, and Islam require women to cover their bodies and limit their movements and activities. The sexes are largely segregated. The lure of women's sexuality is essentially considered irresistible to men. Rape is blamed on lapses in women's adherence to social rules. Even when no such lapse is involved, in some cultures, the raped woman may be made to marry the rapist, or to bring such dishonor to the family that she must be killed by her own male relatives. If it is women's irresponsible lust that is responsible for unplanned and unwanted pregnancies, pregnancy and motherhood, which should be valued, become just punishments for the licentious woman.

What about the psychology of the pregnant woman herself? Of course, women absorb and struggle with the sexual attitudes and mores of their own cultures.[53] There is no evidence that women just want to enjoy sex without wanting or taking on the responsibilities of motherhood, that they do not desire or respect motherhood.[54] In fact, most women have abortions because they have great respect for the responsibilities of motherhood. They feel that the decision to continue a pregnancy should take into account the effect on their existing responsibilities, and that they should give birth to a child only when they have maximized the resources—educational, social, financial—they can bring to its care.

Some women oppose abortion in theory but choose to terminate pregnancies they experience as untenable under their current circumstances. At many clinics where abortions are performed, demonstrators stand outside with signs depicting babies in utero and dismembered fetuses, shout at incoming patients that they are going to murder their babies, and attempt to approach and 'counsel' them against abortion. Physicians who work in these clinics report that some demonstrators take them aside and request abortions for themselves, to be performed outside regular clinic hours so that the other demonstrators do not see them. After their abortions, they resume their places demonstrating outside the clinic. This is not necessarily an example of hypocrisy, but rather of the psychoanalytic 'vertical split'—one part of the psyche opposes abortion on religious grounds, and feels not only justified, but compelled, to oppose it, but another, simultaneously, concludes that a particular, personal pregnancy must be terminated. This dual dynamic may help to explain the discordance between the frequency with which women terminate abortions and the attitudes they express to friends and family, in public, and in opinion polls.

Thus, public attitudes toward abortion, as reported in polls, are misleading.[55] It is essential to know precisely what questions were asked, in what order, and in what context. Most polls offer stark alternatives, sometimes skewed in favor of prohibitions: should abortion be permitted in all circumstances/at all stages of pregnancy or only under conditions such as rape and incest? In fact, people's attitudes toward abortion are complex, nuanced, and context dependent. The same individual who endorses a more or less severe prohibition on abortion may well, if the question is put another way, agree that no one but the pregnant woman herself, knowing her own circumstances, can determine whether it is a good idea for the pregnancy to continue. Opinion polls claiming to demonstrate that women oppose abortion are belied by the greater than 30% incidence of abortion, and, in turn, influence women contemplating abortion; it may be difficult to take an action that you are told that most people oppose.

Expressed attitudes also reflect a superficial resolution of unconscious contradictions. More people apparently believe that an embryo or fetus is a person and that abortion is murder than believe abortion should be illegal in cases of rape or incest. But why should it be acceptable to destroy a fetus/person because it was conceived via rape or incest? This logical lacuna reveals the underlying attitude that being forced to continue a pregnancy is a punishment for a woman's voluntary participation in sexual intercourse; if the participation was not voluntary, the punishment is not necessary, and she need not continue the pregnancy.

ABORTION AND YOUTH

Responses to overly simplistic questions do not allow for consideration of other logical inconsistencies. For example, the reflex answer to the proposition that pregnant adolescents be required to get permission from, or to tell, their parents before being allowed access to abortion is that adolescents are not mature enough to consider the pros and cons of abortion and that their parents have a right, even an obligation, to be involved in or control the decision. But consider the adolescent pregnant from incest or rape by a family friend or relative, the adolescent in an abusive family, the adolescent who realistically anticipates severe punishment or exclusion from the family as a result of her pregnancy. Consider most particularly the fact that the adolescent who is prohibited from having an abortion allegedly because of immaturity will, in a few months, undergo labor and delivery and assume full responsibility for a newborn baby.

The scientific arguments about adolescents' cognitive and emotional capacity to make this decision became somewhat confused because those advocating for parental intervention laws adduced the evidence of adolescent immaturity brought forward by neuroscience experts urging courts and legislatures not to try and punish adolescents for serious crimes as they do adults. Recent publications have clarified the distinction.[56] Adolescents lack adult impulse control and are therefore vulnerable to impulsive criminal behavior. Adolescents do not lack adult capacity to consider alternatives and make decisions like abortion, which cannot be carried out impulsively.

Among decisions about medical interventions, abortion is not a complex one; abortion carries an extremely small risk of morbidity (physical and psychological) and mortality, especially as compared with a continued pregnancy and childbirth, for an adolescent. There is no evidence that abortion causes significant mental illness in adolescents, just as it does not in adults.[57] Adolescent childbirth and parenting are associated with a variety of negative biopsychosocial consequences as compared with abortion during adolescence.[58,59]

THE RIGHT NOT TO BECOME PREGNANT

The defunding of Planned Parenthood is only 1 aspect of barriers to contraception. In the United States, 10.3 million women have had a partner who tried to make them pregnant against their will or who refused to use a condom. More than 2 million women have become pregnant as a result of rape by an intimate partner. Religiously affiliated health systems and work places also have prohibitions against the provision of, or offering insurance for, sterilization and contraception, leaving otherwise insured women fearful of unwanted pregnancy and/or struggling to find the money for these services. Movements to allow over-the-counter oral contraceptives, or allow pharmacists to prescribe them, are a step in a positive direction.[60]

FETAL PERSONHOOD

Another barrier to abortion, and invitation to coercive treatment of pregnant women, is legislation designating the fetus, embryo, or even the fertilized egg as a person, with all the rights of a person. This of course makes abortion murder. In medical terms, pregnancy does not begin until a fertilized egg implants in the uterine wall. The so-called morning after pill, which can be effective up to 72 hours after unprotected intercourse, prevents implantation, but is considered an abortifacient by those who consider a fertilized egg to be a human being. Some states require that a woman undergoing an abortion after a designated gestational age undergo medically unnecessary, possibly deleterious, general anesthesia, with the scientifically refuted rationale that the fetus will otherwise experience physical pain.[61]

The starkest evidence of the denial of human rights is the treatment of pregnant women. As a result of anti abortion activists who assert that embryos and fetuses are persons with all the rights of persons, some women are forcibly and legally subjected to obstetric interventions to which they object, and others are punished for child abuse or child murder for behaviors during pregnancy. These behaviors include suicide attempts, the use of illegal substances, and attempts to abort with medication obtained via the Internet. Pregnant women who are brain dead as a result of injury or disease, who had previously expressed objections to being kept alive if they should succumb to such a condition, and whose families want them to be allowed to die, have been kept on artificial life support until the fetus is deemed viable and is delivered surgically.[10,62,63]

Of course, it is not easy for health professionals to stand by in situations when they believe that they could intervene to protect or save an unborn baby—but they have no right to invade a woman's body or limit her freedom. The American Psychiatric Association and the American College of Obstetricians and Gynecologists have considered the ethics and impacts of these situations and have taken carefully reasoned official positions opposing forced interventions and punitive approaches to pregnancy as well as barriers to abortion and mandated physician statements and techniques.[64–66]

The concept of fetal personhood poses a major danger to women's rights and women's health. The overwhelming majority of women who become, and decide to remain, pregnant are highly invested in the welfare of their unborn children. Setting up a legal conflict between woman and fetus disparages that investment and reduces the woman with individual civil rights to an incubator for a potential person.

ANTIABORTION LEGISLATION AND THE CONSEQUENCES FOR WOMEN'S MENTAL HEALTH

The controversy over abortion in the United States is unique in magnitude, public attention, motivation, and outcomes. Abortion has become a political issue eclipsing many other issues with more impact on national and global benefits and dangers.

With respect to abortion and other reproductive issues, the United States Supreme Court has often shown itself to be out of touch with both the scientific facts and the realities of women's lives. The Supreme Court's *Roe v Wade* decision of 1973 is considered to be the fundamental protection for abortion rights in the United States. The decision has some limitations. It was decided on the basis of privacy rights rather than on reproductive rights. It ordered that states could not enact laws that imposed "undue burdens" on access to abortion before viability. Over the ensuing years, states passed, and the Supreme Court refused to overturn, laws that imposed serious burdens: waiting periods, medically unnecessary interventions, scripted misinformation, outdated and medically deleterious dosage regimens for abortion medications, and rules for abortion doctors and clinics that forced many to close. More than 2500 laws restricting abortion have been introduced in state legislatures during the past 5 years. State laws criminalizing physicians who perform abortions have also been passed.[67]

In the United States, federal funding of abortion services is prohibited by the Hyde Amendment. In addition to women unable to pay for their abortions, this prohibition affects women in the armed services, who may have access only to federally funded care because of military assignments. The Guttmacher Institute reports that, as of March 1, 2016, 11 states restrict coverage of abortion in private insurance plans. Forty-five states allow individual health care providers to refuse to participate in abortions, and 42 states allow health institutions to refuse. Seventeen states mandate preabortion counseling including medically inaccurate statements about abortion, namely, that it causes breast cancer or mental health disorders or that the fetus feels pain. Twenty-eight states mandate a waiting period; one-half of these make it necessary to make 2 trips to the facility. Twenty-five states require that an adolescent obtain parental permission to have an abortion.[68,69]

Both legislation and Supreme Court decisions contain language contravening the evidence of the major medical experts and organizations in the country and mandating unprecedented and unparalleled interference with physician's patient care. Late-term abortions, which are extremely rare and generally performed when the fetus has been found to have defects incompatible with extrauterine life, are most safely performed using the extraction technique; the fetal presenting part emerges from the birth canal before the abortion is completed. State legislation labeled the process the horrific 'partial-birth abortion.' Despite the protests of the American College of Obstetricians and Gynecologists that this procedure is safest for the mother, the Supreme Court upheld a law forbidding it.[67] Antiabortion activists have used the derogatory label for abortions performed earlier in pregnancy as well.

In 2015, a group of antiabortion activists made surreptitious videotapes at Planned Parenthood clinics and falsified the tapes so that they seemed to show clinic personnel selling fetal tissue. Members of the group have been indicted criminally. However, the notion that abortions are being performed so that clinics can profit from the sale of fetal tissue has taken hold. A doctor has been murdered by an individual claiming his intent was to protect baby parts. A congressional committee has subpoenaed the records of a University of New Mexico research project involving donated fetal tissue, demanding and planning to publish identifying information about every person present and/or participating—despite the clear evidence that this unnecessary information will put their lives at risk—also to protect potentially aborted fetuses. This process is being protested as this article is being written. Similarly, the association between Planned Parenthood clinics and abortion in the public, and legislators' minds, has resulted in the defunding and closure of many such clinics, depriving poor women of the contraceptive and general health care, which actually constitute the majority of clinic services.

The US Food and Drug Administration, in 2016, after considering the evidence, simplified the approved regimen for medical abortion.[70] The governor of Arizona signed a bill mandating the use of the previous protocol days before the new Food and Drug Administration guidelines went into effect. This law, like many others, reintroduces the question of privacy into the reproductive rights debate. Monitoring requirements and proscriptions requires intense, ongoing scrutiny of medical records; a requirement for reporting is, in fact, another element of some legislation.

With regard to parental involvement in the abortion decisions of their minor children, the Supreme Court has ruled that parental involvement can be mandated by states as long as there is a provision for a process called a 'judicial bypass.' Thus, a girl who does not wish, or is afraid, to inform her parents that she plans to terminate a pregnancy can go before a judge and assert both the reasons she wishes to have an abortion and evidence of her decisional maturity and/or independence from her parents. This process requires that a girl, first, knows about it, and then is able to locate the correct court and the days and hours it is in session, absent herself from her school or job or parents' home, and master the anxiety nearly anyone experiences in anticipation of an appearance in court. The decisions of courts in these proceedings vary widely from state to state.

The Supreme Court has upheld the prerogative of health systems and facilities to refuse to provide reproductive services in the name of religious freedom.[14,71–73] Religious freedom in the United States was meant to allow everyone to practice, or not to practice, the religion of their choice. Currently, religious freedom is used to allow practitioners of 1 religion to withhold services or rights with which they do not agree, from those of other religions. As of 2016, 1 in every 6 acute care hospital beds is in a Catholic-controlled hospital. In 10 states, more than 30% of hospital beds are in Catholic hospitals, and there are 46 such hospitals that are the sole provider of hospital care in their geographic areas. Catholic health systems require staff to formally agree that they will not even provide information about either contraception or abortion. This prohibition includes mental health professionals, and conflicts with our obligation to learn a patient's reproductive history, intentions, and needs. Consider, for example, the outpatient or inpatient who is pregnant as the result of hypersexual behavior while floridly manic, the patient who becomes pregnant while on large doses of antipsychotics, or the profoundly depressed patient not well enough to care for herself or a baby.

As mentioned, a Catholic hospital will allow a woman to die rather than terminating her pregnancy. Should a female patient in a Catholic hospital request that she undergo sterilization after Cesarean delivery so as to avoid both future pregnancies and the need for another surgical procedure, her request will not be granted. Thus, a woman who has not had success with contraceptive methods must live with the fear of unwanted pregnancy. Catholic hospitals claiming to provide comprehensive care have no legal obligation to inform patients or prospective patients of these restrictions.

The stigma and misinformation surrounding postcoital contraception and abortion has caused many nonreligiously affiliated hospitals to refuse to perform abortions. Public discovery that abortions are being performed are likely to result in demonstrations and a variety of attempts to withdraw the hospital's funding or close it entirely. National law allows anyone in a hospital or clinic who opposes abortion to refuse to participate in it in any way. This allowance leads to situations in which there is no anesthesiologist, nurse, physician, or other staff member necessary to the performance of an abortion.

The so-called morning after pill, or Plan B, is levonorgestrel, which is simply an increased dosage of a common oral contraceptive, effective for up to 3 days after unprotected intercourse. This medication is now approved for over-the-counter purchase—if the product is stocked at the store where the woman looks for it. In some communities, a pharmacy or pharmacist who does offer 'Plan B' may be stigmatized and intimidated. The notion that a woman, who is under time constraints because the medication has diminishing efficacy over time, can simply find another pharmacist to dispense the medication is unrealistic. Her request for the medication reveals her recent sexual activity, which is now known to the pharmacist and to any other staff or customers within hearing distance. Thus a medication that could prevent unwanted pregnancies is not widely available. Wal-Mart, the only pharmacy in many communities, and a major national pharmaceutical source, refuses to stock this medication.

On June 27, 2016, the Supreme Court announced a major milestone in abortion law. The court struck down the Texas law requiring physicians doing performing to have hospital admitting privileges and abortion clinics to meet the building requirements of surgicenters. What is particularly important is the grounds upon which the decision was made. The court defined 'undue burden' for the first time as the imposition of restrictions on abortion that are not supported by medical or scientific evidence, replacing the appellate court decision that laws may be based on "rational suspicion," even in the face of contrary medical evidence.

COUNTRIES OUTSIDE THE UNITED STATES

The World Health Organization proclaims access to all aspects of reproductive health care as a basic, universal human right. Around the globe, the nations where abortions are safe, legal, and available have the lowest incidence of abortion, and unsafe abortion in countries where the procedure is illegal are a, or the, major cause of maternal mortality. Efforts to make abortion legal and available have been successful in a growing list of countries. Before Uruguay legalized abortion, a group of medical professionals and advocates successfully instituted a program gracefully reconciling a nearly total legal abortion ban with the provision of information and care that saved many lives.[74] Health care professionals refrained from performing or advocating for abortion, but informed pregnant patients about the safe use of abortifacient medication they could obtain outside the health care system, and offered safe follow-up both to patients who abort and those who decide to remain pregnant.

SUMMARY: THE NEED FOR FURTHER RESEARCH

We have ample data about the mental health effects of abortion, both completed and denied. There is evidence that the fear of criminal prosecution deters some pregnant women from seeking care for substance or alcohol addiction. We do not have data about the impact of contraception denied or unaffordable, or forced obstetric interventions, or incarceration for behaviors while pregnant. What is the impact of being considered unable to make a decision about a pregnancy without a waiting period or a mandated ultrasound examination? Of being given misinformation about abortion? Of being subjected to surgery against one's will? Of being forced to continue a pregnancy that threatens one's health? Of being forced to continue a pregnancy that will result in the delivery of a severely handicapped infant, or one that will soon die? Of being considered to have fewer rights as a human being than an embryo? There are data about the mental health effects of racial discrimination; being treated as less competent or less worthy, being denied civil rights, because of race, is highly detrimental to mental health. So must be losing civil rights because one is or may become pregnant.

ACTION

Given that reproductive rights are essential to women's mental health; that nearly one-third of women patients in the United States will have or have had an abortion in their lifetimes; and that misinformation, including government-mandated misinformation, is rife, with negative consequences; it is incumbent on mental health professionals to:

- Obtain full reproductive histories from our patients;
- Discuss and destigmatize contraception and abortion;
- Suggest that appropriate patients obtain emergency contraception in advance, to have on hand;
- Inform patients, the public, and policy makers of the facts; and
- Advocate for policy and legal changes to protect women's health.

REFERENCES

1. Inchley J, Currie D, Young T, et al. Growing up unequal: gender and socioeconomic differences in young people's health and well-being. Health Behaviour in School-aged Children (HBSC) study. International report from the 2013/2014 survey. Health Policy for Children and Adolescents, No. 7 WHO Regional Office for Europe.
2. Sonfield A, Hasstedt K, Kavanaugh ML, et al. The social and economic benefits of women's ability to determine whether and when to have children. New York:

Guttmacher Institute; 2013. Available at: http://www.guttmacher.org/pubs/social-economic-benefits.pdf.

3. World Health Organization. Reproductive, maternal, newborn and child health and human rights: a toolbox for examining laws, regulations and policies. World Health Organization; 2014. p. 106.
4. Erdman JN, DePineres T, Kismodi E. Updated WHO guidance on safe abortion: health and human rights. Int J Gynecol Obstet 2013;120:200–3.
5. American Psychiatric Association. Position on family planning. Washington, DC. Am J Psychiatry 1973;131(4):498. Reaffirmed, 2007.
6. American Psychiatric Association, Washington, DC. Position statement on abortion. Am J Psychiatry 1979;136:2.
7. American Psychiatric Association. Position Statement: The Right to Privacy. Reference document No. 910007. Washington, DC: American Psychiatric Association; 1991.
8. American Psychiatric Association. Position Statement on Legislative Intrusion and Reproductive Choice, Official Action. Washington, DC: American Psychiatric Association; 1991.
9. American Psychiatric Association. Abortion and women's reproductive health care rights. Am J Psychiatry 2010;167:6, reaffirmed 2014.
10. Paltrow LM, Flavin J. Arrests of and forced interventions on pregnant women in the United States, 1973-2005: implications for women's legal status and public health. J Health Polit Policy Law 2013;38:299–343.
11. Weinberger SE, Lawrence HC III, Henley DE, et al. Legislative interference with the patient-physician relationship. N Engl J Med 2012;367:1557–9.
12. Merton AH. Enemies of choice: the right-to-life movement and its threat to abortion. Boston: Beacon Press; 1981.
13. Uttley L, Khaikin C. Growth of catholic hospitals and health systems. Geneva (Switzerland): MergerWatch; 2016. Available at: http://www.mergerwatch.org/storage/pdf-files/Growth-of-Catholic-Hospitals-2013.pdf.
14. Cohen IG, Lynch HF, Curfman GD. When religious freedom clashes with access to care. N Engl J Med 2014;371:596–9.
15. State of Indiana. HB 1337, 2016.
16. Maxson P, Miranda ML. Pregnancy intention, demographic differences, and psychosocial health. J Womens Health (Larchmt) 2011;20(8):1215–23.
17. Chakraborty A, McKenzie K. Does racial discrimination cause mental illness? Br J Psychiatry 2002;180(6):475–7.
18. Fernando S. Racism as a cause of depression. Int J Soc Psychiatry 1984;30:41–9.
19. Karlsen S, Nazroo JY. The relationship between racial discrimination, social class and health among ethnic minority groups. Am J Public Health 2002;92(4):624–31.
20. Krieger N. Discrimination and health. In: Berkman L, Kawachi I, editors. Social epidemiology. Oxford (United Kingdom): Oxford U Press; 2000. p. 36–75.
21. Modood T, Berthoud R, Lakey J, et al. Ethnic minorities in Britain: diversity and disadvantage. London: Policy Studies Institute; 1997.
22. Devereux G. A Study of Abortion in Primitive Societies: a typological, distributional, and dynamic analysis of the prevention of birth in 400 preindustrial societies. Review edition. New York: International Universities Press, Inc.; 1976.
23. Riddle JM. Contraception and abortion from the ancient world to the renaissance. Cambridge (MA): Harvard University Press; 1992.

24. Brodie JF. Contraception and abortion in nineteenth-century America. Ithaca (NY): Cornell University Press; 1997. p. 254. ISBN 0-8014-8433-2. OCLC 3769974.5.
25. American College of Obstetricians and Gynecologists. Abortion: resource overview. Washington, DC: ACOG; 2015.
26. Pew Research Center. Religion and public life. Religious groups' official positions on abortion. 2013. Available at: http://www.pewforum.org/2013/01/16/religious-groups-official-positions-on-abortion/. Accessed March 6, 2017.
27. Damian CI. Abortion from the perspective of Eastern religions: Hinduism and Buddhism. Rom J Bioeth 2010;8(1). Available at: http://www.bioetica.ro/index.php/arhiva-bioetica/article/view/149/227. Accessed March 6, 2017.
28. Sedgh G, Singh S, Shah IH, et al. Induced abortion: incidence and trends worldwide from 1995 to 2008. Lancet 2012;19:625–32.
29. Sedgh G, Bearak J, Singh S, et al. Abortion incidence between 1990 and 2014: global, regional, and subregional levels and trends. Lancet 2016;388(10041): 258–67. Available at: http://www.thelancet.com/journals/lancet/article/PIISP140-6736(16)30380-4.
30. Lundberg LS, Pal L, Gariepy AM, et al. Knowledge, attitudes, and practices regarding conception and fertility: a population-based survey among reproductive-age United States women. Fertil Steril 2014;101(3):767–74.
31. Kirkman M, Rosenthal D, Mallett S, et al. Reasons women give for contemplating or undergoing abortion: a qualitative investigation in Victoria, Australia. Sex Reprod Healthc 2010;1(4):149–55.
32. Glander SS, Moore ML, Michiellutte R, et al. The prevalence of domestic violence among women seeking abortion. Obstet Gynecol 1998;91:1002–6.
33. Russo NF, Denious JE. Violence in the lives of women having abortions: implications for public policy and practice. Prof Psychol Res Prac 2001;32:142–50.
34. Silverman JG, Decker MR, Reed E, et al. Intimate partner violence victimization prior to and during pregnancy among women residing in 26 U.S. states: associations with maternal and neonatal health. Am J Obstet Gynecol 2006;195(1): 140–8.
35. Miller E, Jordan B, Levenson R, et al. Reproductive coercion: connecting the dots between partner violence and unintended pregnancy. Contraception 2010;81(6): 457–9.
36. Foster DG, Steinberg JR, Roberts SC, et al. A comparison of depression and anxiety symptoms trajectories between women who had an abortion and women denied one. Psychol Med 2015;45:2073–82.
37. Biggs MA, Steinberg JR, Roberts SC, et al. Mental health diagnoses 3 years after received or being denied an abortion in the United States, 105. Am J Public Health 2015;105:2557–63.
38. Major B, Cozzarelli C, Cooper M, et al. Psychological responses of women after first trimester abortion. Arch Gen Psychiatry 2000;57(8):777–84.
39. Munk-Olsen T, Laursen TM, Pedersen CB, et al. Induced first-trimester abortion and risk of mental disorder. N Engl J Med 2011;364:332–9.
40. Adler NE, David HP, Major BN, et al. Psychological responses after abortion. Science 1990;248:41–4.
41. Major B, Appelbaum M, Dutton MA, et al. Report of the American Psychological Association Task Force on Mental Health and Abortion. Washington, DC: APA; 2008. Available at: http://www.apa.org/pi/wpo/mental-health-abortion-report.pdf.
42. Dagg PK. The psychological sequelae of therapeutic abortion—denied and completed. Am J Psychiatry 1991;148:578–85.

43. Royal Colleges of Physicians. Induced abortion and mental health: a systematic review of the mental health impact of induced abortion. London: RCP; 2011.
44. Cougle JR, Reardon DC, Coleman PK. Depression associated with abortion and childbirth: a long term analysis of the National Longitudinal Survey of Youth cohort. Med Sci Monit 2003;9:105–12.
45. Coleman PK, Coyle CT, Shuping M, et al. Induced abortion and anxiety, mood, and substance abuse disorders: isolating the effects of abortion in the national comorbidity survey. J Psychiatr Res 2009;43:770–6.
46. Major B, Mueller P, Hildebrandt K. Perceived social support, self-efficacy, and adjustment to abortion. J Pers Soc Psychol 1990;59:452–63.
47. Cozzarelli C, Major B. The effects of anti-abortion demonstrators and pro-choice escorts on women's psychological responses to abortion. J Soc Clin Psychol 1994;13:404–27.
48. Steinberg JR, Finer LB. Coleman, Coyle, Shuping, and Rue make false statements and draw erroneous conclusions in analyses of abortion and mental health using the National Comorbidity Survey. J Psychiatr Res 2012;46:407–9.
49. Kessler RC, Schatzberg AF. Commentary on abortion studies of Steinberg and Finer(Social Science & Medicine 2011;72:72-82) and Coleman (Journal of Psychiatric Research 2009;43:770-6 & Journal of Psychiatric Research 2011;45:1133-4). J Psychiatr Res 2012;46:410–1.
50. Rowlands S. Misinformation on abortion. Eur J Contracept Reprod Health Care 2011;16(4):233–40.
51. Stotland NL. The myth of the abortion trauma syndrome. JAMA 1992;268:2078–9.
52. Stotland NL. Abortion: facts and feelings. Washington, DC: American Psychiatric Press; 1998.
53. Major B, Gramzow RH. Abortion as stigma: cognitive and emotional implications of concealment. J Pers Soc Psychol 1999;77:735–45.
54. Moore AM, Singh S, Bankole A. Do women and men consider abortion as an alternative to contraception in the United States: an exploratory study. Glob Public Health 2011;6(Suppl 1):S25–37.
55. Lipka, M. Pew Research Center online. June 27, 2016. Population attitudes towards abortion.
56. Steinberg L, Cauffman E, Woolard J, et al. Are adolescents less mature than adults? Am Psychol 2009;64(7):583–94.
57. Pope LM, Adler NE, Tschann JM. Postabortion psychological adjustment: are minors at increased risk? J Adolesc Health 2001;29:2–11.
58. Leppalahti S, Heikinheimo O, Kalliala I, et al. Is underage abortion associated with adverse outcomes in early adulthood? A longitudinal birth cohort study up to 25 years of age. Hum Reprod 2016;31:2142–9.
59. Henshaw SK, Kost K. Parental involvement in minors' abortion decisions. Fam Plann Perspect 1992;24(5):196–207, 213.
60. Yang YT, Kozhlmannil KB, Snowden JM. Pharmacist-prescribed birth control in Oregon and other states. JAMA 2016;315:1567–8.
61. Lee SJ, Ralston HJP, Drey EA, et al. Fetal pain: a systematic multidisciplinary review of the evidence. JAMA 2005;294:947–54.
62. Pollitt K. Pro: reclaiming abortion rights. New York: Picador; 2014.
63. Pollitt K. Abortion and punishment. NY Times 2016.
64. Committee opinion number 664, American College of Obstetricians and Gynecologists. Refusal of medically recommended treatment during pregnancy. Washington, DC: ACOG; 2016.

65. American Psychiatric Association. Position Statement on Legislative Intrusion and Reproductive Choice, Official Action. Washington, DC: American Psychiatric Association; 2013.
66. Tuerkheimer D. How not to protect pregnant women. NY Times 2015.
67. ACOG Statement Regarding Abortion Procedure Bans. October 9, 2015.
68. Guttmacher Institute. State policies in brief: an overview of abortion laws as of March 1, 2016. Washington, DC. Available at: www.guttmacher.org. Accessed January 26, 2017.
69. Greenhouse L. The abortion map today. NY Times 2016.
70. Greene MF, Drazen JM. A new label for mifepristone. N Engl J Med 2016;374: 2281–2.
71. American College of Obstetrician and Gynecologists. Committee Opinion no. 385: the limits of conscientious refusal in reproductive medicine. Obstet Gynecol 2007; 110(5):1203–8. Available at: http://www.acog.org/Resources-And-Publications/Committee-Opinions/Committee-on-Ethics/The-Limits-of-Conscientious-Refusal-in-Reproductive-Medicine.
72. Sonfield A. Learning from experience: where religious liberty meets reproductive rights. Guttmacher Policy Review 2016;19(1):1.
73. American College of Obstetricians and Gynecologists. Open letter to Texas legislators: get out of our exam rooms (press release). Washington, DC: ACOG; 2013.
74. Adams P. From Uruguay, a model for making abortions safer. NY Times 2016.